POWER PACING

FOR INDOOR CYCLING

By Kristopher Kory
and Tom Seabourne, PhD

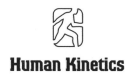

Human Kinetics

Library of Congress Cataloging-in-Publication Data

Kory, Kristopher, 1964-
  Power pacing for indoor cycling / by Kristopher Kory & Tom
Seabourne.
      p.   cm.
  Includes bibliographical references.
  ISBN 0-88011-981-0
  1. Cycling--Training   2. Physical fitness.   3. Physical fitness-
-Psychological aspects.   I. Seabourne, Thomas.   II. Title.
  GV1048.K67   1999
  613.7'11--dc21   98-45940
                                                                     CIP

ISBN: 0-88011-981-0

Portions of this book were adapted from the *Keiser Power Pacer Instructor Training Manual*.

Acquisitions Editor: Martin Barnard; **Developmental Editor:** Laura Hambly; **Assistant Editors:** Leigh LaHood and Laura Majersky; **Copyeditor:** Patricia Fortney; **Proofreader:** Andy Smith; **Graphic Designer:** Nancy Rasmus; **Graphic Artist:** Tara Welsch; **Photo Editor:** Clark Brooks; **Cover Designer:** Jack Davis; **Photographer:** Tom Roberts, unless otherwise noted; **Printer:** United Graphics

Human Kinetics books are available at special discounts for bulk purchase. Special editions or book excerpts can also be created to specification. For details, contact the Special Sales Manager at Human Kinetics.

For more information on workshops and ordering videos, Kris Kory Bike Bands, or other products call 941-417-8931 or e-mail kkpacing@mediaone.net.

Printed in the United States of America   10   9   8   7   6   5   4   3   2   1

Human Kinetics
Web site: http://www.humankinetics.com/

United States: Human Kinetics
P.O. Box 5076
Champaign, IL 61825-5076
1-800-747-4457
e-mail: humank@hkusa.com

Canada: Human Kinetics
475 Devonshire Road Unit 100
Windsor, ON N8Y 2L5
1-800-465-7301 (in Canada only)
e-mail: humank@hkcanada.com

Europe: Human Kinetics
P.O. Box IW14
Leeds LS16 6TR, United Kingdom
+44 (0)113-278 1708
e-mail: humank@hkeurope.com

Australia: Human Kinetics
57A Price Avenue
Lower Mitcham, South Australia 5062
(08) 82771555
e-mail: humank@hkaustralia.com

New Zealand: Human Kinetics
P.O. Box 105-231, Auckland Central
09-523-3462
e-mail: humank@hknewz.com

We'd like to dedicate this book to all those teachers of health, dance, and fitness out there who spend their lives educating themselves and making a difference in other people's lives by getting up every morning, throwing their tape in the machine, and waking up the world with their instruction.

C O N T E N T S

Power Pacing—one of the hottest trends in the fitness industry—is the ultimate indoor cycling program developed by the fitness experts at Keiser. Whether you're a beginner, an advanced outdoor cyclist, or someone looking to add a little variety to your workouts, *Power Pacing for Indoor Cycling* has all the information you need to improve your total fitness. Enlivened by athletic racing, weightlifting exercises, dance movements, and visualization, *Power Pacing for Indoor Cycling* takes the guesswork out of training. The workouts in this book use all of the muscle groups, providing a nonimpact, full-body workout to increase your cardiovascular endurance and build power. The result will be a strong, sleek body without spending hours in a gym.

You can create a fitness program tailored to your needs with this book's step-by-step explanation of how to modify intensity and vary your workouts. The variety of Power Pacing routines and moves, set to music, can easily be transferred to outdoor cycling and other sports as well. The routines themselves can be done in your home or at the many fitness clubs that offer Power Pacing classes. This variety and adaptability is what makes Power Pacing fun and sets it apart from other fitness trends, which often fail to keep the body and mind inspired.

The proper handgrips, body positions, drill movements, and weight training exercises that are used in the Power Pacing workouts are fully illustrated. You can use these photos for learning and as a quick reference to check form and alignment after you've begun training. We also highlight "Power Points" or training tips we have come across in our own experiences, giving you a head start on your path to looking and feeling better.

In chapter 1 we show you how to custom fit your bike, whether it's a Keiser Power Pacer or another brand. You'll also get information on selecting the right clothing and footwear, as well as general guidelines for injury prevention. This information leaves you well equipped to learn the basic positions and drills in the next few chapters.

One of the unique features of Power Pacing is the mind/body experience. Chapter 4, "Psyched for Power Pacing," discusses relaxation, breathing, visualization, and goal setting. With the information in chapter 5 on modifying the intensity of your workouts, you will learn how to fulfill your potential, reaching unimagined levels of power and energy. You will also be able to record and keep track of your progress in the heart rate diary and pacing log chart in this chapter.

Throughout the book there are also a variety of sidebars that offer our real-life experiences, such as how Power Pacing prepared Tom for the Race Across America. They also highlight topics ranging from psychological strategies to competition tips.

Because Power Pacing is both aerobic and anaerobic, many experts believe it is the ultimate workout. Chapter 7 gets you started on this interval training, which will burn fat and build endurance, speed, and recovery. You'll learn actual athletic drills you can combine into a program called Race and Pace, which will help you improve your cardiovascular and cycling skill levels.

Now set it all to music with the rhythmic drills in chapter 8. You'll learn how to combine these drills with different tempos and rhythms to create routines with more variety.

Now that you've got all the basic, athletic, and rhythmic drills down pat, chapter 9 gives you several examples of Power Pacing workouts that you can mix and match for your own heart-pumping, energizing routines. If these aren't enough, seven master trainers are featured in the book, along with their favorite workouts.

Pace and Shape, featured in chapter 10, is a muscle-toning program that includes strength training at the end of your Power Pacing workout. CycleSculpt, a unique and effective cross-training program discussed in chapter 11, uses a new product called the Kris Kory Bike Band that attaches to the bike in many ways for a variety of body-sculpting exercises performed in intervals throughout your entire workout.

Everybody needs a change of scenery now and then, so chapter 12, "Taking It to the Road," lets you take your Power Pacing moves outdoors. Finally, chapter 13 teaches you how to move your workout from the often unpredictable weather of the outdoors to the comfort of your own home.

This book addresses Power Pacing's complete mind/body experience. Once you try it, you'll be hooked!

I would like to express my sincere thanks to my friend and coauthor Tom "the man" Seabourne for all the wit and respect he bestows upon me. My hat goes off to all the certified Power Pacing instructors and club owners out there who have given me so much happiness by allowing me to watch them progress with their successful programs. I'd also like to thank my dear friends and colleagues Tracy Schotanus, Chandra Jones, Jill Watkins, Maureen Hagen, Suya Colorado-Caldwell, Cynthia Groves, Mark Jackson (chief engineer and bike designer), and all the other employees of Keiser Corporation who have given me so much support and kindness. A cheery appreciation goes out to Dennis Keiser and Colin Milner for their brave risk taking in the manufacturing and marketing of such high-quality equipment and for believing in me. Last, and most important, I'd like to thank my parents Bill and Karen, who have always been there for me, keeping life "so real" with their sincere love and the line, "Don't worry, it will all work out!" As always, they were right.

Kristopher Kory

Let me begin by thanking the father of ultracycling, John Marino, who gave me the inspiration to complete the Race Across America; my wife Danese; daughters Alaina, Laura, Susanna, and Julia; and my only son Grant, who rides with me daily. Thanks to my developmental editor Laura Hambly, Human Kinetics Publishers, all of my colleagues at Keiser, and especially to Kris—one of the most street-smart men I know. Finally, I want to dedicate this book to my dad, who recently passed away, and to my mother for her strength in holding everything together.

Tom Seabourne, PhD

ACKNOWLEDGMENTS

PRIMED FOR POWER PACING

You've finally discovered the ultimate workout, and you're no doubt anxious to start reaping the rewards—a strong, sleek, healthy body; enhanced performance; and a healthy mind. There are, however, a few things you need to know before you begin your Power Pacing program. In this chapter you'll learn how to choose a bike and adjust it for maximum comfort. You'll also learn the types of clothing, footwear, and accessories that will result in the best performance. To prepare your body for the workout of your life, we also provide tips on hydration and injury prevention. So before you cue your music, take the time to learn what you need for Power Pacing success.

Choosing Your Bike

Before you can begin logging mile after mile in your Power Pacing workouts, you'll need the most fundamental piece of equipment—the bike! If you're planning to Power Pace at a fitness club, the type of bike you use may already be decided for you. If you're looking to purchase a bike, you'll want to find out which one is right for you. First, you need to know what's out there.

Keiser Corporation manufactures three different types of stationary bikes:

- The Power Pacer—a fixed gear or direct drive stationary bike (see figure 1.1).
- The freewheel bike—a non-fixed gear bike, similar to a regular bike feel (see figure 1.1).
- A recumbent freewheel bike—great for those folks who are not comfortable on an upright bike due to the small seat, or who lack the coordination and strength to maintain an upright position without back support (see figure 1.2). The recumbent freewheel bike allows you to do only seated drills.

The Freewheel Bike

Before you choose, it's important to know the difference between a fixed gear or direct drive stationary bike and a freewheel stationary bike. A freewheel bike allows for a slower workout that requires more power and attention to detail of resistance. When you increase speed on this bike, you must also increase resistance just like on a real road bike. This is similar to changing gears and is so that the flywheel does not get ahead of your pedal stroke. On a freewheel bike you can also coast any time you want since there is no fixed gear system keeping the pedals in motion the way there is on a Power Pacer or direct drive stationary bike.

Individual energy output must equal resistance at all times or you will acquire an uneven pedal stroke on a freewheel bike. A skipping movement is an indication that one component in your spin cycle is greater than the other. If this happens, you must either slow down or apply more resistance to the pedals.

The Freewheel Formula developed by Tracy Schotanus

Energy output + Resistance (without skipping) = Appropriate individual workload

Following this formula will ensure the appropriate workload specific to your individual needs at all times. It is impossible to go too fast without enough resistance on a freewheel bike. In other words, you can't cheat.

The Fixed Gear Bike

Unlike the freewheel bike, the Keiser Power Pacer (or a direct drive stationary bike) has a fixed gear, which means that it doesn't coast

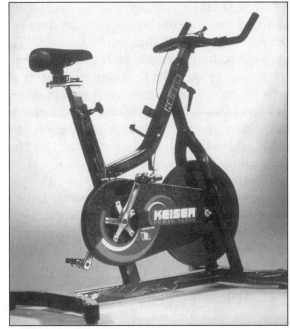

Courtesy of the Keiser Corporation

Figure 1.1   The Power Pacer/freewheel bike.

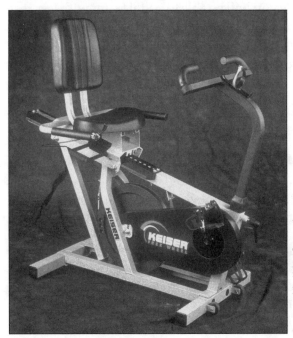

Courtesy of the Keiser Corporation

Figure 1.2   The recumbent freewheel bike.

like a freewheel or road bike. For this reason, it's very important that you understand how to stop the bike—just turn the resistance lever counterclockwise—if your foot slips out of the pedal. The flywheel and crank are fixed so that once you start pedaling a bit of inertia is built up helping you to keep the flywheel turning. It is possible to work speed drills above your normal working speed or cadence on this bike. But beware, uncontrolled speed could be harmful to your joints and connective tissue. Whenever you are on any stationary bike, you should feel as though you are in control and not as though the bike is controlling you. Injury can occur when you do not control your speed.

If you don't have a Keiser bike at home but do have a stationary bike, get it out of the laundry room or garage, dust it off, and try it out. Test it to see if you have a direct drive or freewheel version by pedaling slowly and trying to stop. If the pedals stop immediately and the wheel keeps moving, you have a freewheel bike. Be sure to follow the freewheel formula as described.

If you are looking for a bike that absolutely simulates outdoor cycling and want the freedom to just stop and coast at will, then the freewheel bike is for you. If you are looking to train at speeds higher than those you would normally train at outdoors, the Power Pacer is for you since you will be able to pedal faster with less resistance. This type of training can be very beneficial for a cyclist who is looking to improve his or her speed on the flat road.

Bike Setup

Setting yourself up on the bike is an important part of the ride and helps you to avoid an uncomfortable ride and possible injury.

Seat and Pedal Adjustments

The proper seat height allows you to use your muscles most efficiently and provides you with a safe position for your knees. Always adjust your bike seat while standing on the floor. Never stand up on the pedals to adjust your seat since you may fall off your bike and hurt yourself.

If you have a front-to-rear seat adjustment, place the seat directly over the post before adjusting the height. Then stand next to your bike and bring the seat up to hip joint height. Now flip your pedal over so the cage is on the bottom, mount the bike, and place your heel on the center of the pedal. In this position, with the hips level, the knee should be just slightly bent.

To secure your foot in the standard cage-type pedal (see figure 1.3), flip the pedal around and place your foot into the cage so the ball of your foot is over the center portion of the pedal next to where it attaches to the crank arm. Tighten the strap by pulling up on it, making sure it is not in the safety keeper. Once snug, place it in the keeper and you are ready to ride. When you're done exercising, open the buckle by first pulling it out of the safety keeper and then pushing out on the inside of the tab.

There are many different types of clips and pedals available at your local bike shops. One of the most common types is the SPD combo pedal that has a cage-type pedal on one side and a clip system for attaching an SPD cycling cleat on the other. This pedal is shown in figure 1.4. To release your foot from the clip, just turn it to the side and it will pop out.

If you purchase new pedals for your home bike, remember that the left pedal has reversed threads and must be turned to the right to unscrew it from the crank arm. It is designed this way so the pedal does not unscrew when you're riding.

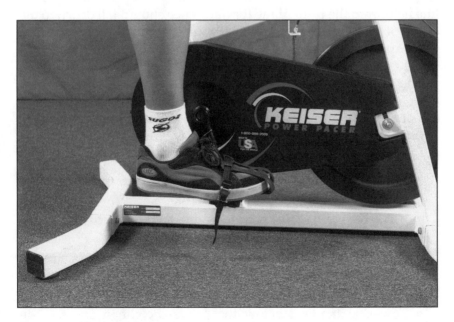

Figure 1.3   Cage pedals.

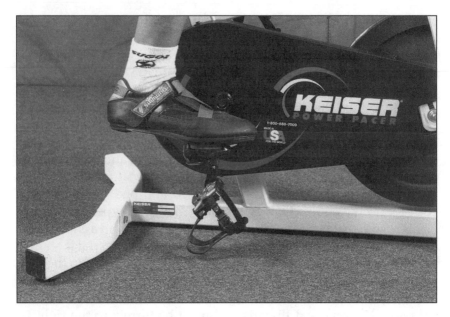

Figure 1.4 SPD combo pedals.

If your bike has a front-to-back adjustment, turn the pedals so the crank arms are parallel to the floor. In the correct position, a plumb line held from the front of the forward knee should fall down to the center of the front of the foot. Adjust your seat forward or back to find the proper position. If the seat is too far forward, pressure may be felt in the knees.

The nose of the seat should be parallel to the floor or slightly elevated to provide the best comfort. You should never feel as if you are sliding forward. Always sit on the back portion of the seat.

A few things to examine after you have set the seat height include the following:

- If you are pointing your toe down when riding, the seat may be too high.
- If you are riding with your knees pointed outward, the seat is probably too low.
- Always push from the center of the metatarsal area of your foot and not from the arch since that could cause cramping and soreness in that soft tissue area.
- Lowering the seat below the proper height in order to do specific isolation work for the gluteals is not recommended. This puts unnecessary strain on the knee joints.

Handlebar Height

The handlebars should always be in a high, comfortable position for beginners, as shown in figure 1.5. As a general rule, in the basic riding position and in hook grip, you should be able to maintain a neutral spine position without strain in the upper back while keeping the elbows soft. In this position, adjust the handlebar height up or down to provide the most comfort. Once you have determined the proper handlebar height, be sure that the handlebar tightening pin is pointing either up or down, not to the side, since a taller person riding the bike may rub a knee on it if he or she moves forward too much when riding. This pin can be adjusted without affecting its tightness by simply pulling it out away from the bike and turning it.

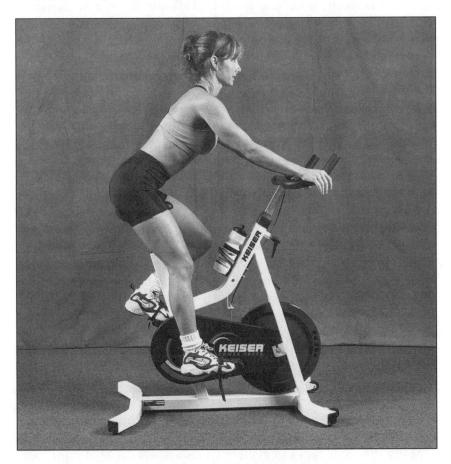

Figure 1.5 You know your handlebars are the right height when you can maintain this correct body position.

> **Power Point**
>
> If you are an avid outdoor cyclist, you may want to match the adjustment of the seat and handlebars of your Power Pacer to fit the dimensions of your outdoor bike. In this way you can work identical muscles from similar angles to enhance your racing performance.

Flywheel Belt Adjustment

Keiser bikes have a buckle or tightening bar on the front that allows anyone to personalize the resistance adjustment for his or her own strength level and weight. With the resistance lever in the no resistance position, pull the strap through the end of the buckle or bar, making sure there is about a quarter-inch of slack at the bottom of the flywheel. Put a small amount of tension on the bike and see if the tension strap activates the flywheel while pedaling. If not, pull a little bit more of the strap through the buckle or bar and try again. With the resistance lever at the full resistance position, you should be able to stand up and barely move the pedals, if at all. If the lever slips back, tighten the wing nut or screw on top of the resistance lever by turning it clockwise. If that doesn't help to provide tension, check to see that the strap is in the flywheel groove at the bottom of the flywheel and that it is attached to the spring at the end of the resistance cable.

Clothing and Footwear

Now that you have your bike and know how to set it up, let's discuss what to wear during your workout.

The best type of shorts to wear is padded cycling shorts designed to be worn without underwear. These can be purchased at most bike shops or sports outlet stores. Be aware that not all cycling shorts are created equal. Turn the shorts inside out to make sure there is no seam down the middle of the padding. Seams can become uncomfortable when riding.

G-string or thong-type leotards and underwear tend to be uncomfortable. Running shorts are also uncomfortable since the elastic tends to rub against your skin as you move your legs. If you want to wear running shorts with the built-in undergarments, wear tight-fitting sport shorts or leggings under them to prevent rubbing.

Many different types of cycling shoes are available at your local bike shops. If you have a specific type of bike pedal, you will need a specific type of cleat for your shoes. Mountain biking shoes tend to be very comfortable for indoor cycling, as are good, strong cross-training shoes. The only shoes to watch out for are those that will not give you enough support when you stand, such as an old pair of running shoes or sandals.

Power Point

Always make sure that your shoelaces are tied very short, tucked under your laces, and/or double tied since the force of pedaling will often cause them to come undone and get caught in the crank arm of the bike.

Now that you've picked out a pair of padded shorts and some sturdy shoes, consider investing in the following accessories to make your workouts go even more smoothly:

- Have a towel handy since this is a very sweaty sport.
- Bike gloves help with calluses and slippage on the handlebars. Look for gloves that have rubber gripping on them.
- A gel seat cover provides a bit of extra cushioning when starting out.
- Have a good tape or CD player to play your favorite music.
- A heart rate monitor will allow you to watch your heart rate and stay in the preferred zones.

Power Point

Heart rate monitors are vitally important to your safety. Do not monitor your heart rate solely by the way you feel since it is very difficult to determine your heart rate when performing this type of workout.

Preparing Your Body

To be on the safe side, it is always advisable to start slow and listen to early warning signals of overworking, such as loss of breath, discoloration of the face, weak legs, and nausea. If you have led a sedentary life for a long period of time, are over 35, have high blood pressure or a heart condition, have had recent surgery, are pregnant, or are on any heart rate regulating medications, consult with a physician before starting this or any cardiovascular program.

Hydration

Adult bodies are approximately 65 percent water and need to stay hydrated while exercising in order to maintain proper levels of performance. Drink one to two cups of fluid 20 minutes before you begin your workout so you are well hydrated. Have a sports bottle filled with cold water and drink small sips every two to four minutes while cycling. You should easily finish 16 ounces of water in a 45-minute workout. In hotter climates drink more since you will be perspiring at a much more rapid rate than normal.

If you are hypoglycemic, diabetic, pregnant, or plan on exercising longer than 40 minutes, seek advice from your physician since you may need to be drinking some type of carbohydrate drink when working out to help regulate your blood sugar levels.

Injury Prevention

Proper mechanics are vital to avoiding the onset of discomfort. Always make sure you are set up properly on the bike and using correct alignment and body mechanics. Most common discomforts can be alleviated easily by using proper technique and taking a few precautions.

The number one complaint from indoor cyclists seems to be soreness where the hips make contact with the seat. There are four main reasons why this happens. The first is not wearing the proper clothing, as we discussed earlier. The second is pedaling too fast without enough resistance, which causes your hips to bounce on the saddle. The third is improper positioning of your body on the saddle. The nose of the saddle should be level with the back of the seat or slightly elevated. Your ischial tuberocities, the bones under your pelvis, should be able to make contact with the rear portion of the seat. If you ride too far forward, the nose or center part of the saddle will be pressing against your soft tissue causing bruising and possible injury. Finally, it is important that you ride only 20 minutes during the first couple of workouts to allow for a gentle break-in period.

Chafing and sweating can lead to saddle sores. These are a type of crotch infection that can start out as a small pimple and may become hard, red, and inflamed. Protect yourself by wearing the correct clothing and immediately removing wet cycling shorts when you are finished training. Since most problems are bacterial in nature, cleanse your body with an antibacterial soap. If after three or four days saddle sores do not disappear, seek professional help. Cycling clothes that have been worn should be washed and dried thoroughly before using them again to prevent bacteria buildup.

Low back, neck, wrist, foot, and knee pain are also common complaints when first starting out. Be sure you are always set up properly on the bike and using correct hand and body positioning. Following are symptoms and possible solutions to different types of pain. They are intended as suggestions only. If any of these discomforts linger, it is always a good idea to seek advice from a physician for proper diagnosis.

• Low back pain can result from tucking the hips under and not maintaining a neutral spine. If you start to experience low back pain, avoid twisting at the waist while on your Power Pacer; lifting both legs simultaneously; or engaging in any rapid arm movements, unsupported forward flexion, or hyperextension.

• Neck pain can be caused by rounding your back and not retracting your shoulder blades.

• Wrist or forearm pain can be caused by not maintaining a proper line between the forearm, wrist, and hand. When people get tired, they often break at the wrist.

• Foot cramping can result from riding with your feet too far up inside the cage or gripping with your toes when you ride.

• Knee pain can be caused by improper tracking or having your seat too far forward.

Your Knees

The first thing you may notice on professional cyclists are the large quadriceps muscles just above their knees. The knees themselves are the framework for these engine-like muscles. Hopefully, your knees are in perfect working condition. If they are not, your doctor may actually prescribe Power Pacing as an antidote.

The Framework for Your Engine. Your knees are your Power Pacing pistons. They are also the anatomical pulleys between your femur (thigh bone) and your tibia (shin bone) and fibula (small bone beside your tibia). Your knees are amazing joints, but they are very much exposed. They are on the front of your body and get bumped and banged up. When you fall, you usually land on your knees. In addition, knee joints are shallow; one bone does not fit tightly into another. Consider them similar to hinges.

Yet when you bend your knees to pedal, unlike a hinge, they can rotate too, making them even more complicated. Several muscles extend your knees to allow you to press down on your pedals. These include your four quadriceps muscles, which are your rectus femoris, vastus lateralis, vastus medialis, and vastus intermedius. They are on the front of your thigh.

Studies demonstrate that elite cyclists do little "pulling up" on their pedals when cycling on level ground. These investigations failed to examine sprinting and climbing, however. During Tom's first ultra-endurance race, the SPENCO 500, he was competitive with other racers on the straightaways. But on hills, just about everyone left him in their dust. As he watched them speed by, he noticed that all of them had cycling shoes that clipped to their pedals. He could see their hamstrings and glutes propelling them up the hills. No matter how hard he was pressing down on the pedals with his quadriceps, he could not match their speeds. They were pulling up, using their hamstrings and glutes. Because they were able to use more muscle groups, they rode faster with less fatigue.

Your hamstrings, in the back of your upper leg, generate knee flexion. These muscles include your biceps femoris, semimembranosus, and semitendinosus. They flex your knees so you can pull up on your pedals. Your hamstrings are generally weaker than your quadriceps. If your hamstrings are more than three times weaker than your quadriceps, then you have a muscle imbalance that may precipitate knee problems.

You can evaluate your quadricep-to-hamstring strength ratio using a Cybex machine. Or, after a thorough warm-up, attempt a 1-repetition maximum lift on the leg extension and leg curl machine in your local gym and then quantify your results. Strengthen your hamstrings by doing muscle recruitment drills, which are discussed in chapter 3. Flex your hips at a 90-degree angle by sitting back on your saddle and dropping into your aggressive riding position (described in chapter 2). Without pointing your toes down, feel your hamstrings pull your heels toward your buttocks.

On the inside of your knees, closest to your groin, you have muscles called adductors. Your adductor magnus, adductor longus, adductor brevis, and gracilis keep your knees aligned while pedaling. If your knees have a tendency to bow out, a gentle reminder to contract your adductors will help pull them into proper position.

On the outside of your knees you have abductors. Your tensor fascia latae and gluteus medius pull your leg away from your body. Your adductors and abductors stabilize your movements when you flex and extend your knees on each pedal stroke. A combination of knee flexion, extension, and stabilization from your adductors and abductors enable you to turn tiny circles in smooth, rhythmic revolutions.

When you extend your knees on your pedal stroke, there is a slight lateral rotation of your tibia and femur. This is termed the "home screw mechanism." You may notice a figure S or figure eight motion during each revolution. This may not be cause for worry if adduction of the thigh compensates for the inward rotation of the knee. If the abnormal pattern stems from excess pronation of the foot, however, an orthotic is recommended.

Women sometimes have trouble with their knees because of the width of their hips. A normal Q angle, which is the angle drawn from the outside of your hip down to your knee, is 10 degrees. If the Q angle exceeds 10 degrees, the kneecap becomes unstable. Men and women with bow legs or knocked knees can learn to adjust their cycling frequency, intensity, and duration to prevent knee problems.

Zeroing In on Knee Pain.   Understanding the anatomy of your knees can help you prevent some of the causes of inflammation that some folks experience. Pain on the outside of your knee during your pedal stroke may be aggravated by friction on your iliotibial band. Your iliotibial band is a long, fibrous, tendinous sheath located on the outside of your leg that extends from your hip past your knee. Stretches such as the lower body stretches in chapter 6, anti-inflammatories, and ice may help. Also try lowering your bicycle seat.

Pain behind your kneecap may be the result of chondromalacia, a progressive softening of the patellar cartilage. Cartilage is the cushion between bones. The semilunar-shaped cartilages in each knee, which are called meniscus, act as shock absorbers. To alleviate any pain in the kneecap, pedal with light resistance and try raising your seat. You can strengthen the quadriceps muscle on the inside of your knees by using the muscle recruitment exercises in chapter 3.

If you use heavy resistance or don't warm up properly, you may develop patellar tendinitis. Your patellar tendon, located just below your kneecap, attaches your tibia to your kneecap. When sore, ice your patellar tendon for five minutes, massage it for five minutes, and then repeat this sequence.

Power Point

If you have patellar tendinitis or chondromalacia, do not put heavy resistance on the flywheel. Instead, pedal faster to increase your intensity. This is *your* ride.

Pain on the back of your knees may be bursitis. Three muscles, the sartorius, gracilis, and semitendinosus, meet at the pes anserine. Inflammation occurs here if these muscles rub against one another. Rest and ice may be helpful.

In any case, check with your doctor. He or she will probably ask for a more detailed description of the origin of your pain. You may also be asked to take part in an arthrogram or arthroscopy to get a clearer picture of the reason for your distress.

Listening to Your Body

In addition to monitoring and maintaining proper body alignment and technique, it is also a good idea to take notice of the following: loss of breath, excessively high heart rate, weak legs, discoloration of the face, loss of motor control, nausea, and vomiting. If you exhibit any of these signs, pedal slowly and take small sips of water. If you know you are prone to any of these conditions and you are working out alone, you may want to keep a phone close by with phone numbers handy in case you need to call for help.

You've outfitted yourself with the right Power Pacing apparel and equipment, you know the secrets to quelling discomfort, and you realize the importance of monitoring your body and maintaining good technique. Now you're ready to learn just what we mean by good technique.

HAND AND BODY POSITIONS

As you are learning each of the hand and body positions, pay close attention to the form of each in order to protect yourself from injury. Many hand and body positions can be used for several different drill variations, and a few of them are very specific to the drill you are performing. Change your hand and body positions often so you don't get bored and your body doesn't get too used to one position. Variety is what keeps Power Pacing so interesting; there is always something else to try.

Hand Positions

Ten variations for placing the hands on the handlebars are possible. You should use the most effective hand position for your body position or the type of drill you are performing. Always make sure to maintain a straight line between the hand, wrist, and forearm for proper biomechanics.

Poor alignment of the wrist could cause injury. For example, if you allow the heels of the hand to push down and break at the wrist in the overhand grip, you may be setting yourself up for an overuse injury, such as carpal tunnel syndrome. Your handgrip should always be relaxed with your elbows slightly bent in each position. Never lock them. This will keep the stress off the wrist joint area.

Overhand Grip

In the overhand grip, the heels of your hands should rest gently over the crossbar of the handlebars. Make sure to keep your thumbs on top of the handlebars. This will keep you from gripping the handlebars too tightly.

You will use this hand position for some seated riding drills and when performing the rhythmic drill called seated push-ups, discussed in chapter 8, to strengthen the triceps.

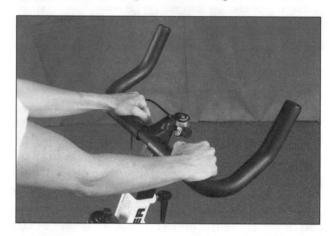

Corner Grip

The heels of your hands should rest gently on the handlebar curves with your elbows facing slightly outward, away from your body.

This grip is used to strengthen the chest muscles when performing seated push-ups.

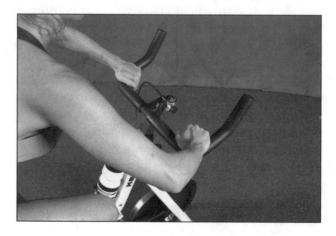

Hook Grip

Place the fleshy part of your hand located between your thumb and first finger in the hook of the handlebar where the parallel bars begin to curve up. While maintaining a loose, relaxed grip, keep your elbows a little wider than shoulder width.

The hook grip is the most common grip, as it is used for many of the seated and standing drills.

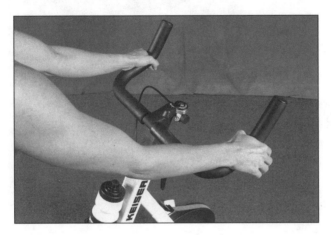

Aggressive Grip

Hold on to the end part of the handlebars where they curve up. Keep your elbows a little wider than shoulder width without resting your forearms on the handlebars. The shoulders should stay behind the elbows. See the photo on page 18.

The aggressive grip is used for the aggressive seated or standing body positions only. This is due to the uncomfortable and biomechanically incorrect position of the wrist when the aggressive grip is used in conjunction with other, "nonaggressive," body positions.

Parallel Grip

With the elbows facing out, internally rotate your wrists with fingers and thumbs facing each other on the inside of the handlebars. Lightly place the heels of your hands on the handlebars without applying any of your body weight. See the photo on page 18.

This grip is used when performing standing dips.

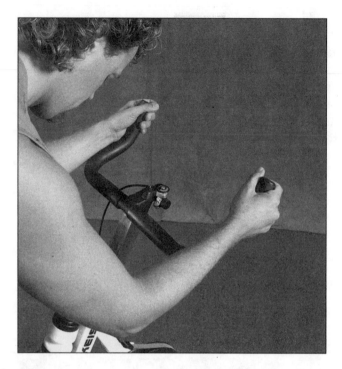

Aggressive grip.

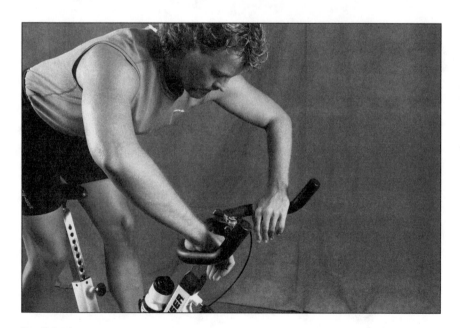

Parallel grip.

Seated Parallel Grip

Slide the heels of your hands up to the highest point of the handlebars with your elbows out and your fingers and thumbs facing inward. This grip is used to perform seated dips.

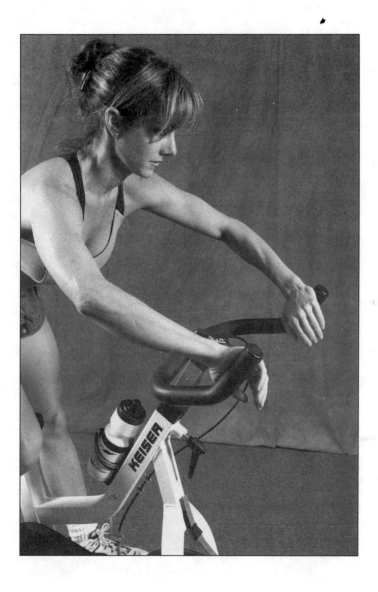

Vertical Jog Grip

Place your fingertips on the overhand grip area of the handlebars. This grip is used when performing the vertical jog drill.

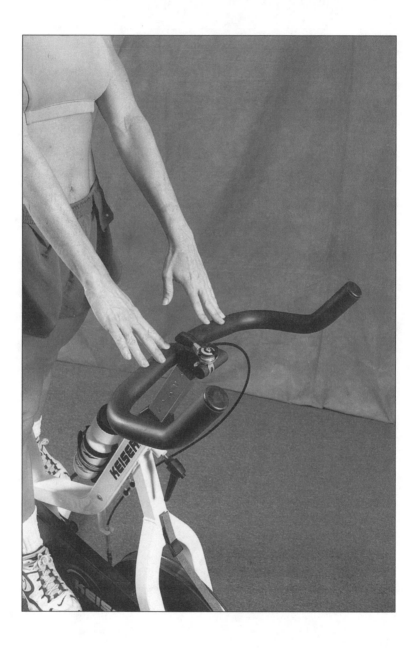

Cupping Grip

Rest the palm area of your hand on top of the end of the handlebars. Be sure that your wrist and forearm are in line with your hand.

This is a great grip for people with long arms and flexible torsos. It can be used for many seated and standing drills, such as a seated climb or a standing climb in a basic riding position.

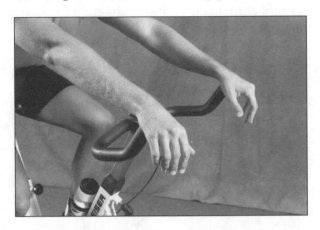

Diagonal Grip

Place one hand in an overhand grip and the other hand in a hook or cupping grip.

The diagonal grip is used when you want to focus on using one lead leg. For example, if you are performing a lead leg drill (see chapter 8) emphasizing the right leg, then the right hand would be forward in the hook grip position.

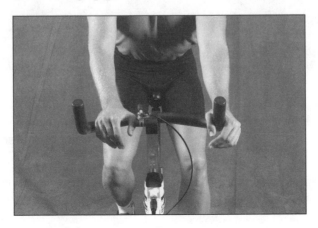

Forearm Lean Grip

Let your elbow and forearm of one arm rest on the handlebar and place some of your body weight onto it. Always remain seated with this grip, and abstain from pedaling.

This grip is used to stabilize the body when performing such exercises as bent-over rows and triceps kickbacks with handweights. It enables the other arm to move the handweight freely and keeps the focus on the upper body.

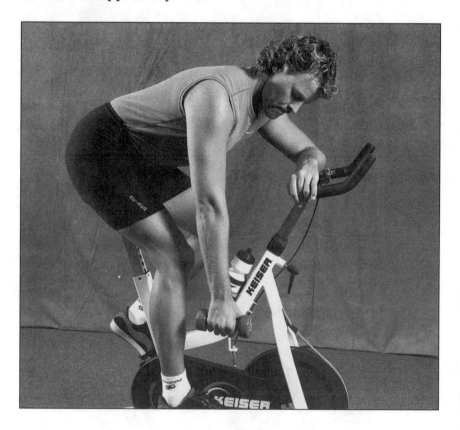

Power Point

Prevent hand and wrist numbness by switching grips often.

With the availability of ten different handgrips, you have a lot of options for keeping your Power Pacing workouts fresh and interesting.

Body Positions

In each of the five body positions, proper biomechanics are vitally important to positioning yourself correctly during your workouts.

Following are three key points to remember in each of these positions, except the reversed basic riding position.

1. Always maintain a neutral spine. This means that you must keep your spine lengthened with a natural lumbar curve at all times. Never tuck your hips under.

2. Keep your shoulders retracted. Never allow your shoulders to raise up by your ears causing you to round your upper torso. This creates a great amount of unnecessary pressure and stress in the neck area.

3. Keep your navel pulled tightly in toward your spine. Your torso needs to be stabilized at all times to avoid stressing your low back. This also helps to work the abdominals throughout your workout.

Seated Upright Position

You will use this first position (shown on page 24) when warming up and also for water breaks. Sit in the saddle with your torso upright and perpendicular to the floor. Your arms should be at your sides.

Basic Riding Position

With your hands on the handlebars in a hook grip, your torso should lean slightly forward at about a 45-degree angle. See page 25.

This position is used for many seated (see page 7) or standing drills. When standing, keep your hips directly over the top of the saddle. Do not move your body forward or lean on the handlebars.

Power Point

You use more muscle groups standing than you do sitting since you are putting your whole body weight onto your legs instead of distributing it between the seat and your legs.

Reversed Basic Riding Position

This position is the same as the basic riding position, except that you will slightly extend your spine and reach your chest up toward the

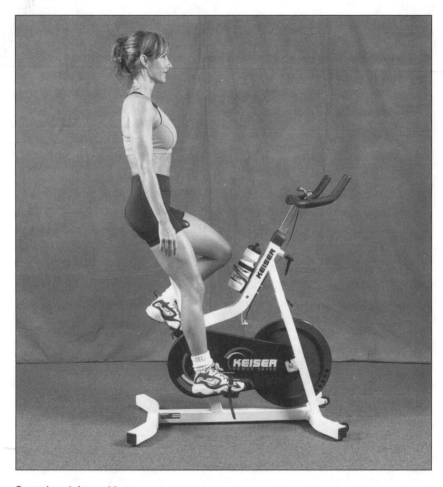

Seated upright position.

ceiling, as shown on page 26. You should feel a slight arch in your back and your rib cage should be spread open in the front.

This is a good position to use when you start to feel yourself bending over too much and rounding your back.

Aggressive Riding Position

The aggressive riding position, shown on page 27, can be done in a standing or seated position. It is the most advanced position; it can be challenging for beginners and people who lack flexibility in their backs and hamstrings. Beginners should pay close attention to their low backs in this position. If you notice that you are feeling too much

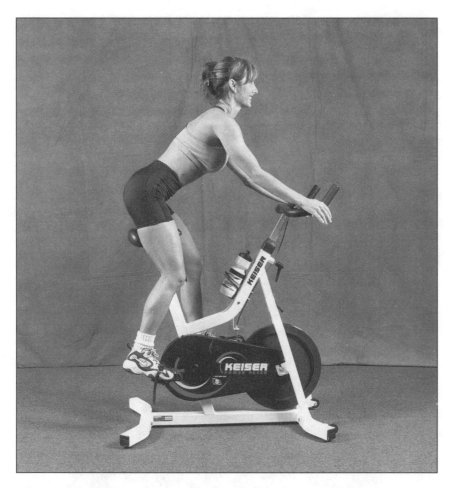

Standing basic riding position.

strain or stress, stay in the basic riding position until you become more fit. Make sure to take some extra time to stretch out your back muscles at the end of your workout. See the stretching segment in the cool-down section of chapter 6 for some back stretches.

Reach your hands out to the aggressive grip and position your spine so it is parallel to the floor. Be careful not to tuck your hips under too much or to put weight on your forearms.

When standing, just slide your hips up and back over the saddle. Do not move your body weight forward onto your hands. In the correct standing position, you should feel a stretch in your hamstrings and a slight concave arch in your low back as you maintain a neutral spine.

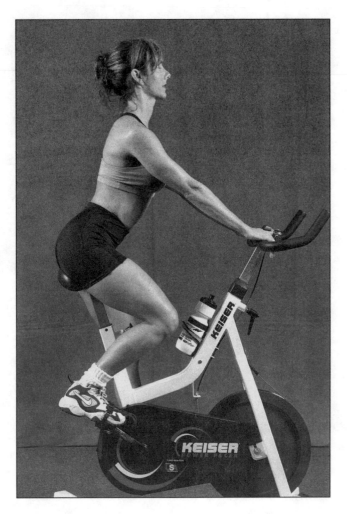

Reversed basic riding position.

Vertical Jog Position

Stand straight up on the pedals in a vertical position as if you were climbing a ladder or walking down the street. Place your hands in the vertical jog grip without leaning forward. See the photo on page 28. This body position is used when performing the vertical jog drill.

Proper hand and body positions provide variety in your workouts to keep you interested while also providing the framework for proper biomechanics when riding. Take time to really watch and feel your form. Position yourself sideways to a mirror and check to see if you are truly maintaining that neutral spine in all positions (except

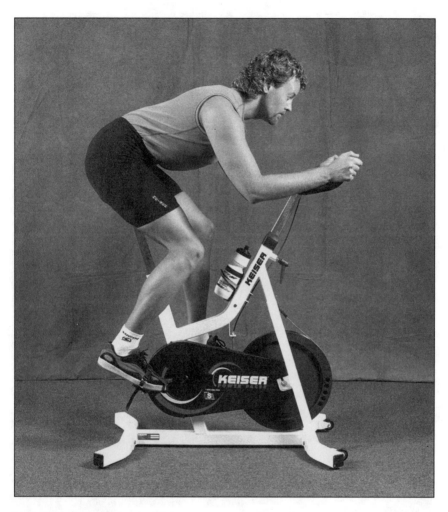

Seated aggressive riding position.

Power Point
Always work on the bike in a square and balanced way maintaining a parallel knee position and keeping your knees angled over your feet. Refrain from moving your hips side to side, which affects the knee joint alignment.

the reversed basic riding position). Use the aggressive riding position to challenge yourself and take breaks by sitting upright. If at any time you notice tension building up in your upper and / or low back, move into the reversed basic riding position to perform an

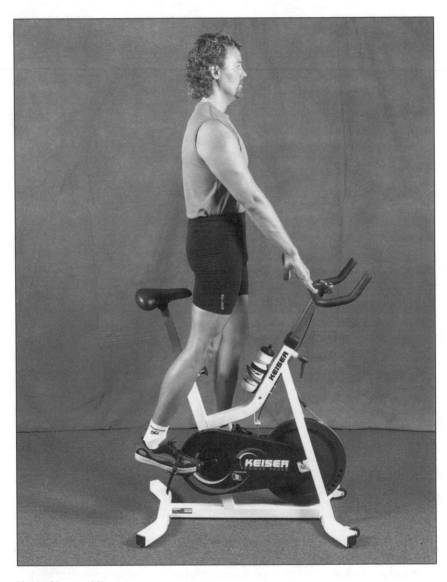

Vertical jog position.

opposition stretch, especially if you have a tendency to round your back when your ride.

Now that you have a good understanding of these positions, move on to chapter 3 and learn how to apply them to the basic drills. Let's get pedaling!

BASIC DRILLS

The basic drills provide the framework for all of the athletic drills, which you'll learn later. Learning how to be proficient in each of the basic drills with regard to proper body positioning, form, and control of your pedal stroke; understanding how to modify the intensity of each drill with the appropriate resistance; and, finally, learning how to combine them will provide you with a fun and effective workout.

Practice the basic drills provided in this chapter so you can progress to more advanced programming. Your body will adjust to the different postures and pedaling speeds. Train with your basic drills often to develop a strong foundation—then you can tackle more difficult Power Pacing techniques.

When you are first learning how to put your cycling program together, you can combine seven basic drills with the hand and body positions in chapter 2 to form the framework of your program.

## CHAPTER 3

SEATED UPRIGHT DRILL

The seated upright drill is performed in the seated upright body position with arms at your sides and light resistance on your bike. Light resistance would be enough tension to feel the belt grab the flywheel. The tension lever will be in different places for different people since their strength levels vary. It is important to keep your pedal speed at a slow, comfortable pace without losing any control of the upper torso.

This is the drill to use when you are warming up at the beginning of your workout and during water breaks.

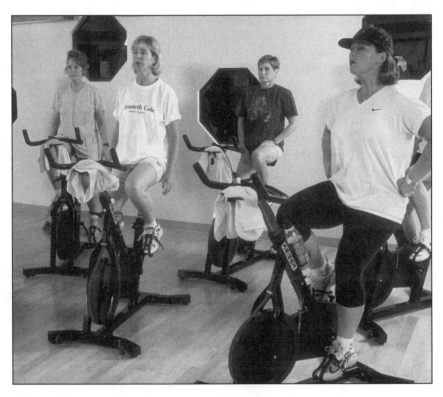

Start out with the seated upright drill to warm up your body.

SEATED CLIMB

The seated climb can be performed in either the basic or aggressive riding position with medium to heavy tension on the bike. Overhand, hook, or cupping grips work best for this drill when you are in the basic riding position. The aggressive grip is, of course, always used in the aggressive riding position.

When performing a seated climb, keep your pedal speed slow to medium and imagine yourself climbing a steep hill while sitting in the saddle. If you feel any discomfort in your knees when performing a seated climb, reduce the tension and make sure you are keeping your knees aligned over your ankles.

Power Point
Use the aggressive grip only when you are in the aggressive riding position.

VERTICAL JOG

The vertical jog drill can be performed two different ways. Both variations are performed standing in the vertical jog body position with medium resistance.

1. Add your resistance and stand up. Then pedal at a slow to medium speed, allowing your body to move up and down like a piston in a car. Always maintain control of the pedal stroke and keep your upper torso stabilized. This is a great variation to use when you don't want to sit down but need a little break.

2. Assume the same body position as above, but keep your body from moving up and down. Your upper torso remains still while your legs pedal away! This is an incredible leg strengthener, and it teaches you how to ride with control. Transfer that feeling of control into all of your standing drills.

STANDING CLIMB

The standing climb can be performed in either the basic or aggressive riding position with medium to heavy tension on the bike. The hands may be in an overhand, hook, or cupping grip. Keep your pedal speed slow to medium, maintaining control of your pedal stroke without allowing your body to bounce up and down.

While performing the standing climb, make sure to keep your hips directly over the seat. As your legs get tired, you will have a tendency to move your hips forward in front of the saddle when you stand, thereby putting unnecessary strain on your knees. By keeping your hips over the seat, your body weight will be concentrated more on your legs than on the handlebars.

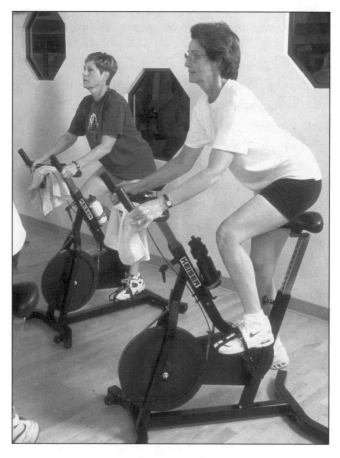

Move into a standing climb to really challenge your leg muscles.

FAST HAMMER

The fast hammer drill simulates a sprint. It can be performed in a basic or aggressive riding position, seated or standing, with your hands in a hook or aggressive grip, respectively.

While pedaling at a quick pace, always use light to medium resistance. A good indication that you do not have enough resistance is when your hips bounce up and down on the seat and you feel a loss of control in your pedal stroke.

Performing a fast hammer in a standing position is extremely advanced since it requires a great deal of control and strength to keep your body positioned properly and to refrain from bouncing.

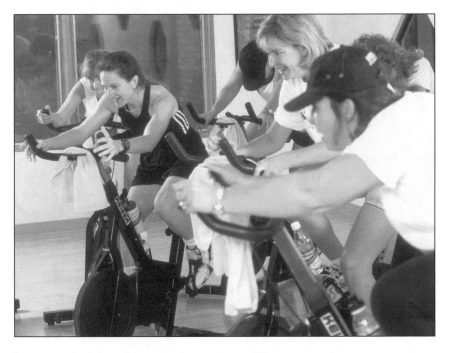

Lower your body into that aggressive position and hammer away!

Power Point

If your hips are bouncing up and down on the saddle, apply more tension or slow down.

MUSCLE RECRUITMENT

The muscle recruitment drill is used to strengthen the leg muscles and help you understand how to use different muscle groups throughout the pedal stroke. Once you understand how to recruit different muscles when cycling, your pedal stroke will become more efficient and your quadriceps will not burn out so quickly.

This drill is performed in a seated basic riding position only. The hands are in an overhand, hook, or cupping grip. Resistance should be medium to heavy.

Following are the three variations of muscle recruitment:

1. The first variation focuses on the quadriceps or top of the upper thighs. Push straight down into the pedal stroke.

2. The second variation focuses on the hamstrings, or the back of the upper thighs. Focus on wiping your feet on the floor as you curl your legs behind you. Do not point your toes down.

3. The third variation focuses more on the gluteals and the back of the hip area. Focus on driving the pedal stroke forward as if you are performing horizontal leg presses or riding a recumbent bike.

FLUSHING

The flushing drill is used to recover. Reduce your tension and allow your legs to just move with ease as you feel your body cooling down. Flushing can be performed in any seated body position using any handgrip you feel comfortable with.

The basic drills should be practiced, practiced, and practiced since they are the most important part of your riding technique. They will be combined in chapter 7 to form the Athletic Training Drills.

Before moving on to creating your workouts, it is important to understand how to use your mind to attain maximum adherence to your workouts, how to stay focused, and how to use breathing to control the intensity of your workouts. Now move on to the next chapter and let's get psyched for Power Pacing!

PSYCHED FOR POWER PACING

Pedaling is more than just turning little circles with your feet. It is important to be relaxed and focused on your bike. This chapter will explain how to personalize your program to pedal according to your needs and the goals that you design for each Power Pacing workout. You will learn to breathe correctly and focus on the proper cues for exemplary riding. Techniques and strategies for talking to yourself effectively, visualizing your pedal stroke, and associating with your muscles will fuel your pedaling power. And when your endorphins kick in, there will be no stopping you!

Relaxation and Mindfulness

Mindfulness is simply concentrating on exactly what you are doing when you are doing it. Can you pedal and think of nothing but your pedal stroke? Most of us can't because we're stressed. Stress has become a chronic problem for many people. The pace of our lives can be so fast that even with such "modern conveniences" as car phones, computers, and fax machines, we still work day and night. Our bodies are able to handle stress, but not all of the time. We must be able to respond to stress and also know how to relax.

Power Pacing is an excellent way to simulate the stressors you face every day and to practice the relaxation you need. For example, a fast hammer stresses your body, while flushing produces profound relaxation. Special mind/body Power Pacing drills allow you to experience a continuum of extremes in a controlled setting. Power Pacing teaches you the flexibility to bend instead of break.

Walking, jogging, or pedaling an exercise bike for 20 minutes reduces stress, but Power Pacing goes a step further. Mind/body strategies, such as imagery and association, provide you with mindfulness both on and off the bike. Mindfulness can help you relax. When you claim you don't have time to relax, that is when you need relaxation the most. Start by learning the relaxation techniques in the following section. Do them *on* your bike, then use the deep-breathing and tension-releasing exercises to help alleviate the stressors you face *off* your bike.

Relaxing on Your Bike

You can relax before, during, and after your ride. Warming up and cooling down require a relaxed demeanor, but it is also important to enjoy muscle relaxation throughout your workout. We're not talking about a collapsed dishrag, but the kind of relaxation that allows you to be alert and focused with each pedal stroke.

In the seated upright position, hold your abdominal muscles in and your shoulders back and down as your low back maintains a natural arch, keeping you in a neutral spine position. Relax your entire body. Become especially aware of upper body tension and let those muscles relax. Allow tension in any part of your body to be released. You cannot force yourself to relax. Relaxation will happen if you clear your mind and glide through your pedal stroke. When your legs relax, you will automatically pedal more easily and efficiently.

Now it's time to focus on your breathing. Pedal slowly and take deep breaths, inhaling through your nose and exhaling through pursed lips. Breathe from your diaphragm instead of your chest. To accomplish this, sit upright and perform a breathing drill. Inhale from your nose, taking five pedal strokes to expand your lungs. Focus on raising your diaphragm. Fill your lower, central, and upper chest, in that order. Then take 10 pedal strokes to exhale through your mouth by lowering your diaphragm.

To combine mindfulness with deep breathing and pedaling, take deep breaths from your diaphragm with long exhalations. Pedal to the beat of the music, focusing on your breathing. When you breathe

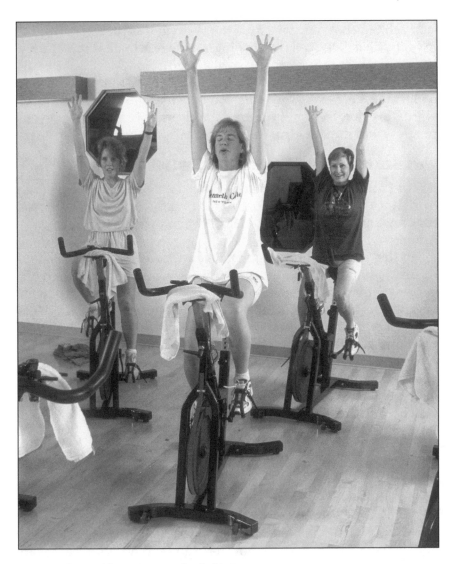

Stretch, relax, and leave your tension behind you.

Power Point
If you are tired, a deep breath can make you more alert.

from your navel area, your diaphragm is activated. This allows you to take deeper and longer breaths, using more of your lung capacity. Double your pedal stroke using the fast hammer drill. Your breathing and heart rate increase. Breathe deeply from your diaphragm so your stomach pouches out. Take in as much oxygen as possible. Imagine oxygen-filled blood cells nourishing your legs. Exhale automatically. Your pedals are flying on their own accord.

Mindfulness gets easier with practice. Similar to Power Pacing, mindfulness is a skill. The more you rehearse, the better your focus will be. But don't worry if you are a slow learner. Concern about your progress will impede your improvement.

Personalizing Your Workout

Power Pacing is unique in that each person, according to his or her own fitness level, can personalize his or her workouts. *You* set the resistance and the speed. *You* decide when to challenge your body further and when to relax.

Try this exercise: immerse yourself in Power Pacing. Pedal and relax simultaneously. Your pedal stroke is your mantra. Each rhythmic revolution relaxes your mind and body. Mindfulness is not hard or time consuming, but simply a matter of focusing on each pedal stroke. Let distractions enter one ear and proceed out the other. Continue pedaling and breathing at your individual cadence. Personalize it. The timing is yours, not an instructor's or video's. Once you decide the level at which to perform, let nothing distract or disturb you; just pedal and breathe. If thoughts or sounds interfere, notice them, but let them go.

Keeping the Drive Alive

Motivation to Power Pace comes easy for some; they set goals and pedal until they reach them. Whether you want to lose body fat, tone your muscles, or improve your cardiovascular system, your first step is to decide what you hope to accomplish. Then progress gradually until you meet some of your short-term goals. When you reach your long-term goal, you will deem yourself successful.

Setting Goals

Success is measured in achievement. Reaching lofty goals seems easy for some until we peer behind the scenes. Consider doctors, lawyers, and professional athletes: we sometimes forget how hard they worked in the classroom or on the playing field. Some paid an awesome toll early on and later reaped tremendous rewards.

You, too, have the opportunity to achieve fitness beyond your expectations, and you can enjoy the process. But first you must

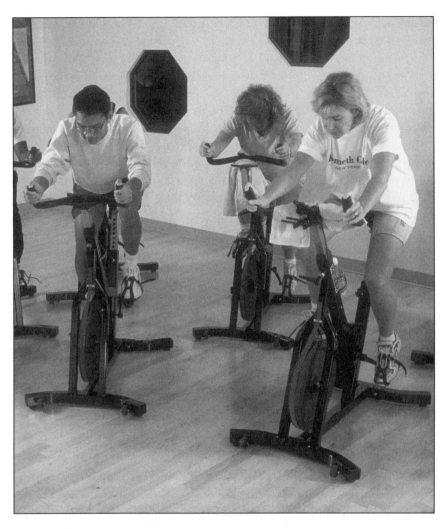

Focus on yourself. Let those around you fade into the background.

prepare. Close your eyes and take a few moments to determine your desires. Make mental notes or write them down. Don't hesitate to explore seemingly unattainable ideals. Nothing is far-fetched. How would it feel to gain strength and endurance and lose weight? Spend a few minutes just before going to sleep mentally preparing for the next day. Try to fall asleep at a reasonable hour and awaken early; each hour brings you closer to your health, fitness, and Power Pacing goals. Visualize yourself enjoying Power Pacing. Feel the energy surging through your body. Sculpt a perfect model of your physique by enlarging your muscles and slicing away fat. Relish the concept of moving toward your ideal self.

After you decide what your long-term goals are, such as gaining strength and endurance or losing weight, you need to set achievable short-term goals that will equip you to tackle your mission. If your short-term goal is to lose body fat, begin training at an easy pace and intensity, and progress gradually. Daily short-term targets inspire you, and early achievements serve as incentive. These small successes will provide endurance for the long haul. Begin with baby steps, and in six months you will become accustomed to your Power Pacing program. Increase your intensity no more than 5 percent for a given workout. If you are too vigorous, your body and mind will revolt. With proper planning, however, you can discipline yourself to do almost anything.

Do you Power Pace to fit into your jeans? Although this may be one of your goals, don't fret about losing weight. When your mind is ready, your body will follow. Lao-tzu, an ancient Chinese philosopher, said, "Building your body can be achieved only when your mind has been disciplined."

No worthwhile goal is simple. Prepare for distractions and obstacles. Motivation waxes and wanes, and there will be pitfalls. Your body will find reasons to get off the bike. The secret is to convince yourself that Power Pacing is play. How can spending time straddling a bicycle seat be pleasurable? It's fun if you know when to start and when to finish. Start by setting guidelines as to how much time you want to devote to Power Pacing. A Power Pacing workout may be completed in 20 minutes. If you do find yourself lacking motivation, page through *Power Pacing for Indoor Cycling* and use our words and photos for encouragement and inspiration.

Turning pedals is half your training. The other half is mental. Tap into your goals. As minute-to-minute, day-to-day, month-to-month, and year-to-year goals are reached, seek new ones. Maintain your program until it is routine, then alter it so you don't get bored. If you

---

Power Point

Power Pacing increases strength, endurance, and flexibility and decreases your chances for heart disease, diabetes, and hypertension. It increases your energy and metabolism and decreases your body fat, mid-afternoon lethargy, and mood swings. An afternoon of lounging can't beat a spirited Power Pacing workout!

always look forward to Power Pacing, you will never burn out. Priorities may conflict, so be flexible. Set aside a few minutes several times a week. Once Power Pacing is a habit, it's easy. Whether preparing for cycling competition, improving health, getting fit, or reducing stress, no two Power Pacing workouts are alike because each fulfills a different promise of perfection.

Mental Preparation

How much time do you spend Power Pacing each week? Is the mental aspect of Power Pacing important? If you answered yes, then how much time do you spend mentally preparing to Power Pace? Try the following two-minute technique, followed by the goal-directed affirmations.

Two-Minute Mini-Imagery Technique

1. Close your eyes and relax (10 seconds).
2. Breathe from your diaphragm. Focus on your breathing (30 seconds).
3. See, feel, and experience yourself pedaling (40 seconds).
4. Enjoy a sensation of perfect balance, control, and heightened speed (20 seconds).
5. Let these feelings reinforce themselves (10 seconds).
6. Slowly open your eyes (10 seconds).

Goal-Directed Affirmations

1. Power Pace daily with a clear, uncluttered mind. When you get on your bike, leave all distractions behind.
2. Spend a few moments pedaling in goal-directed relaxation.
3. Turn the pedals and visualize your ideal self.
4. Zero in on the goals you've set for yourself, such as becoming faster, healthier, or stronger.
5. Adjust your goals to your capabilities.
6. Visualize your goals and the training required to reach them.
7. Evaluate whether you have reached a goal, then set a new one.

The Endorphin High

There are no bad workouts; some are merely more or less intense than others. A single session does not make or break your regimen. The hundreds of Power Pacing programs are what matter. Enjoy deep levels of relaxation and concentration while pedaling unrestrained.

Power Pacing opens capillaries and stimulates the production of morphine-like painkillers called endorphins. Power Pacing junkies can reach an "endorphin high." Endorphins attach to nerve cell receptors in your brain. The receptors combine with chemicals blocking the transmission of pain. A feeling of joy is the result. Research by a foremost authority on endorphins, Atko Vuru, PhD, demonstrated that to experience endorphins you must exercise at 76 percent of your maximum heart rate. Some people experience an endorphin high in 30 minutes. For others it may take as long as two hours or more, and 10 percent of the population never feel it. Some Power Pacers do not feel the high at all and some only after two or more hours.

If you mount your Power Pacer and you feel sluggish, pedal a few strokes. Generally, following the warm-up, your endorphins kick in and you gladly complete your workout. The hardest part is getting started. Lee Berk, PhD, showed that endorphins can be produced simply by anticipating activity, so spend time daydreaming about your next drill. Close your eyes prior to each song. Take 30 seconds to see, feel, and experience the approaching routine. Do not permit negative thoughts. If you are in the middle of your visualization and think, "I'm tired, I'm not going to finish," then immediately change your thought to, "STOP, I was tired, but I'll complete my drill and feel great."

Beginning Power Pacing

The following objectives will help you start, and stick to, your workouts.

Month 1: Make your Power Pacing a habit.

1. Do not miss any workouts during your first month.
2. Clear your schedule to be sure of no conflicts.
3. If you dread pedaling, tell yourself you can quit after a month.
4. Reward yourself after each Power Pacing workout with a cold drink.
5. After a month of Power Pacing, evaluate your progress.

Month 2: Enjoy your training.

1. Go out of your way to introduce yourself to other cyclists.
2. Set training goals based on your potential.
3. Make it a point to ask a Power Pacing instructor about your progress.

Month 3: Put your heart into your training.

1. Each time you Power Pace, work on a specific goal (e.g., speed, intensity, flexibility).
2. Work on your weaknesses as well as your strengths.
3. Give 100 percent of yourself to each of your Power Pacing workouts.
4. Practice the finer points and details of your Power Pacing drills.

No Pain, No Gain

The origin of Power Pacing discomfort is not the issue, controlling it is. Instead of discussing the misery of saddle sores, we will discuss alleviating pain by releasing the tension, slowing your pedal stroke, or stopping pedaling. However, remember that if you never challenge yourself to 30 more seconds on a pyramid climb, you will never ascend the fitness ladder. Accept pain for what it is and handle it. Face discomfort and learn about it, and Power Pacing won't seem severe.

Change how you think about pain. Acknowledge it. Be objective. The burning in your quadriceps on hill sprints is from lactic acid. Muscles generate lactic acid during your entire Power Pacing workout, but your kidneys and liver absorb it. Depending on your cadence and resistance, lactic acid is either generated or removed. The faster and harder you pedal, the more lactic acid you produce. Pedaling with less effort helps to disperse lactic acid from muscles into your bloodstream to be recycled to produce more energy. When you reach your anaerobic threshold, however, the lactic acid production exceeds the removal rate and the acid remains in your muscles, causing pain. This pain can be avoided simply by remaining below your anaerobic threshold.

The sensation of pain depends on how you think and feel about it. Because pain is sensory, emotional, and cognitive, the pain messages that reach the brain can be controlled. The mind can magnify pain or sublimate it. Pain signals scream so loudly that they drown out rational thought. Change those howls of agony to shouts of joy. Pain often protects you from serious injury. There is a distinction between pain you should deal with and pain that says "Stop." The first few Power Pacing workouts are the most intense. Muscle fibers split and joints ache. You can choose to interpret these signals as debilitating or change them to wonderful sensations of Power Pacing success.

Your ability to handle burning in your thigh muscles is what sets you apart. Approach Power Pacing with courage. Deal with it on your terms. Handle pain one step at a time. Preparing for pain helps you to endure it. Power pacing enthusiasts revel in lactic acid. Those last three drills may seem severe, but the brain transforms them into joy.

Psychologists claim humans need some pain in order to function. We seek an optimum level of pain, a level we can handle. Goal-directed pain may be endured. When Tom rode 458 miles in the 24-hour Ironbutt ultramarathon cycling race, he experienced pain the whole time. Rather than succumb, he acknowledged pain's presence and focused on his rock and roll audiotape. Power music was his painkiller.

Pain is an "in the moment" experience. Try reading this sentence while pedaling a fast hammer for five minutes. See which gets your attention. Pain protects you from injury. While experiencing the doldrums of the Race Across America, Tom promised he would never do ultradistance cycling again. A week after completing the race, however, he was training for next year's event. Feeling good and reaping the benefits of racing across America far outweighed the discomfort.

Association and Dissociation

Association and dissociation are mental techniques that help you to perform better on your bike. Association is feeling your muscles working. When you associate, you focus on fibers splitting and blood rushing into your muscles.

Dissociation is the opposite of association. Instead of concentrating on the muscles that are working, you distract yourself. You can use music, drills, or simple daydreaming to pull yourself away from discomfort. Pedal slowly. Gradually pick up your speed. You are not lethargic or agitated. Do not try. Trying slows you down. Instead, provide a relaxed effort. Gauge your rpms.

Nerves send lactic acid pain messages to the spinal cord, which delivers them to the brain. Sean McCann, sport psychologist at the

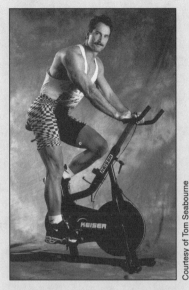

Courtesy of Tom Seabourne

Tom Seabourne's Muscle Recruitment Mind/Body Class

This is a great drill because it not only gets you relaxed, it puts you in the perfect workout "zone." By focusing on tension and relaxation of your body, you'll forget all distractions. This is a drill that really helps me relax before competitions.

Record the following and use it as an instructor-guided drill:

Close your eyes. Pedal smoothly and gently with no resistance on the dial. Place your right hand on your chest and your left hand on your stomach. Breathe from your diaphragm so that only your left hand moves. Like an infant. No cares or worries. Just listening to your bike, the music, and my voice. Nothing to bother or disturb you. Focus on the circular pattern of your pedal stroke. If any unwelcome thoughts enter your mind, let them flow in one ear and out the other. Relax more and more deeply.

Now, slowly open your eyes. Rest your hands in the overhand grip. Press your chest toward your handlebars in slow motion: 1, 2, 3, hold. Slowly bring your body back to an upright vertical position. Feel your triceps working. Relax. Notice the difference between the tension and relaxation. Downstroke to the beat of the music.

Shrug your shoulders toward your ears. Hold it: 1, 2, 3, relax. Notice the difference between the tension and the relaxation. Let your feet find the beat.

Bring the palms of your hands together at chest leve!. Press tightly: 1, 2, 3, relax. Notice the difference between the tension and relaxation. Your knees are pistons, let them go.

Extend your right arm up as if raising your hand. Make a fist with your right hand. Imagine that it has been encased in lead. It is growing heavier, and heavier, and heavier. It is getting so heavy that it is beginning to fall back down toward your side. As it falls, the muscles in your upper body are becoming more relaxed. As they become more relaxed your mind relaxes, and you find yourself more open to suggestions. Allow the suggestions to provide you the best workout of your life. Thirty more seconds. Fast hammer!

Now increase to heavy tension on the flywheel. Press the balls of your feet through the floor and focus on your quadriceps. Feel the blood surging into your quads. Your muscles are burning and your fibers are splitting. Take the tension off and flush. Notice the difference between the tension and relaxation.

Now click your dial up to heavier tension and focus on the back of your legs as you imagine wiping gum off the bottom of your shoes, as you curl your heels toward your buttocks. You rarely get to work these muscles. Focus on your hamstrings. Feel them lengthen through the full range of motion of your pedal stroke. Remove the tension and flush. Notice the difference between the tension and relaxation.

Let your hips settle back on your saddle. Click up to heavy tension and press forward from your heels as if performing a leg press. Concentrate on your gluteals. They become rock-hard with each extension. Remove the tension and flush. Notice the difference between the tension and relaxation.

Resume the seated upright position and continue flushing. Take a drink. Place your hands in the hook grip and lengthen your spine by assuming the reversed basic riding position. Hold for three seconds: 1, 2, 3, relax.

Tom is a two-time National Tae Kwon Do champion; the author of five books on fitness, health, and stress management; and a top ten finisher in the grueling Race Across America. He is also the holder of five ultra-endurance national cycling records and the 1995 Ironbutt champion.

Olympic Training Center in Colorado Springs, Colorado, teaches athletes to use key words and imagery to reinterpret pain signals more positively. Pain diminishes when you call it something else. Simonton, MD, says to picture your lactic acid pain as a glowing orange ball. Then see your body fending off the pain (for example, visualize the glowing orange ball disappearing).

A Power Pacer may describe discomfort as enjoyable, but others may never truly understand the description. Don't say, "The race is almost over and I can quit." Give everything you have until you pedal your last revolution. Let your mind dictate the movement of your muscles. Learn and practice the art of association. Focus exclusively on your effort. You must be in control of your pain. Dissociate during your Power Pacing warm-up. Associate on speed bursts.

Try the following: place your palms five inches from each other. Imagine heat energy flowing from one palm to the other and back. Similarly, you can send blood to your legs to power your pedal stroke. Dissociate from the boredom of long hill sprints by picturing yourself in a peaceful scene. Imagine yourself skating effortlessly up a mountain. Dissociation is setting the mind apart from the body.

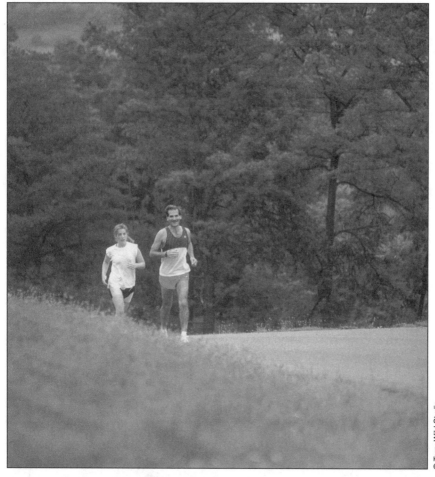

© Terry Wild Studio

Natural surroundings help many runners get through a run. Make your next workout easier by picturing yourself cycling through this same scenery.

A recent study by David Roth, PhD, on 150 recreational runners demonstrated that dissociation provided them with more vigor both during and after their runs. The top eight dissociation topics included relationships, housework, building homes, life problems, natural surroundings, job and career, recent hurt or anger, and finances. Plenty of world-class athletes and entertainers dissociate from the regularity and pain of their training and performance. You can pedal through a multitude of drills in what seems like only a few minutes if you dissociate by focusing on the music. Or you can associate by recruiting every fiber of your hamstrings to pull through on your pedal stroke. Changing your mind about discomfort can change your body.

Try the following exercise: monitor the mechanics of your fast hammer. Knees over toes. Pistonlike. No mashing (mashing is when you press too hard on the pedals, which sometimes leads to knee and hip problems). Add resistance. Stand. Pull from your hamstrings on the upstroke. Your hamstrings are thick, strong cables. The lactic acid burn is intense. Dissociate. Breathing is your only interest. Sway from side to side with each pedal stroke. Stay on the beat. When your attention disengages from your breathing, simply try to refocus on it. Let your pedals follow the music.

Quitting is usually the first option when confronted with fatigue and discomfort. But if your goal is to succeed, sometimes it is useful to persevere. Expect to get through discomfort. Teach your body to handle discomfort a little at a time. Reach deep inside and ask a little more of yourself for each Power Pacing workout.

Psychological Strategies

Power Pacing requires a narrow, internal focus of attention, as opposed to the broad, external focus a football quarterback must possess. Choose to associate with your body by feeling every aspect of the pedal stroke. Visualize fibers splitting and blood pumping to your quadriceps, hamstrings, gluteals, gastrocnemius, and soleus. While associating with your muscles, you will find that random thoughts will enter your mind in the form of self-talk. Talk to yourself nicely.

Self-talk takes the form of positive affirmations, such as, "Pedaling fast is easy." These self-verbalizations raise arousal levels. Although your arousal level may increase, relax your muscles. With relaxation comes speed and efficiency. Relax and notice if upper body muscles are wasting precious energy.

Controlling Fatigue and Discomfort

The following is a tool to help you reach your Power Pacing goals. Use these affirmations when cycling becomes unbearable.

1. Fatigue exists in your mind.
2. You can beat fatigue and discomfort.
3. Pushing yourself through discomfort will lead you to your goal.
4. An increase in "the burn" is a signal that you are nearing the finish line.
5. Be objective about the burn and fatigue. Observe it. Enjoy it.
6. You have the power to control your thoughts.
7. Your mind is capable of focusing on only one thing at a time.
8. When the lactic acid burn and pedaling fatigue become unbearable, let your focus change.
9. Let yourself become part of the music.
10. Enjoy focusing on your beat; the discomfort will disappear.

Power Point
Positive self-talk will give you the drive you need to complete your workout.

A simple way to increase your relaxation and pedal speed is to use mental imagery. Picture yourself Power Pacing. Several studies suggest that when we visualize ourselves training, nervous impulses are sent down the proper neuromuscular pathways to stimulate muscle fibers, enhancing speed and performance.

Relax and pedal while chatting with your teammates and navigating imaginary roads. There is no competition. Front-runners have no worries of comrades falling off the pace. A rebellious upstart may quicken the tempo, but she is ignored by the pack. The pelaton begins and finishes together. Nobody flaunts speed, career status, or education. Racial differences do not exist. You finished. You're a winner.

Buddhists repeat mantras, and yogis assume postures. For centuries, Eastern mystics have been searching for enlightenment.

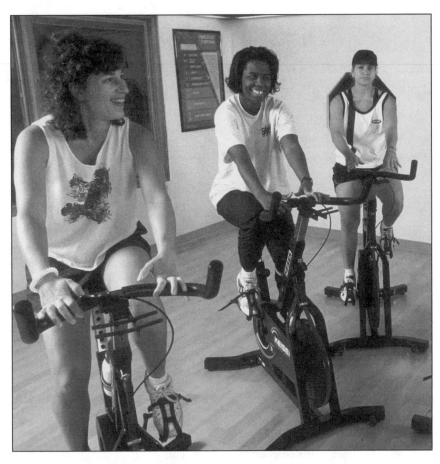

Log imaginary miles as you and your teammates go for an easy ride.

Maharishi Mahesh Yogi brought Transcendental Meditation (TM) from India to the United States. Mihalyi Czicksentmihalyi termed this state of relaxed concentration *flow*. Harvard cardiologist Herbert Benson, guru of mind/body medicine, transformed TM into the Relaxation Response. His research demonstrated that the Relaxation Response lowered blood pressure and increased health and well-being. Recently, Benson discovered that cycling was as effective as the Relaxation Response for escaping into an altered state of consciousness. Focus your mind and body and find your zone—pedal tiny, little circles.

INTENSITY TRAINING

Knowing how hard to Power Pace is important. Sometimes you pedal too vigorously and discover you are overtraining. But if you don't pedal fast enough, you may not achieve your fitness and performance goals. Be sure to read this chapter carefully; it discusses training zones, maximum heart rates, and individual goal setting in order to achieve maximum results.

Realizing Your Aerobic Potential

If your goal is to be fit and healthy, cardiovascular (CV) exercise can be an important step. Your CV system includes your heart, lungs, circulatory system, and tiny capillaries that supply oxygen and energy to your muscles. CV exercise can combat obesity, high blood pressure, and glucose intolerance. Twenty minutes of Power Pacing three or four times a week is the most effective way to improve the efficiency of your CV system. As your CV system improves, you burn fat more efficiently. Your body will be transformed into an aerobic furnace.

If you are Power Pacing in your target heart rate zone, your exercise is aerobic. Your blood delivers a continuous supply of oxygen to your working muscles. Pedaling at a constant pace for 10 minutes, as during a long hill climb, is an example of aerobic exercise. Find your "steady state" by pedaling at a constant pace, slow enough so that you can carry on a conversation. You might be huffing and puffing a little, but you should not feel a lactic acid burn. During aerobic exercise oxygen is your energy source, allowing you to pedal for long periods.

Power Pacing at a consistent speed for as little as 10 minutes can improve your cardiovascular endurance. A great training effect of

Power Pacing is that your resting heart rate will generally slow down. In fact, Power Pacing may strengthen your heart, providing for a greater stroke volume to pump more blood through your body with each beat. You may notice an increase in energy, and you will be able to work longer and harder without fatigue.

Finding Your Zone

When starting to organize your workouts, it is important that you understand how your body responds to the training drills that you

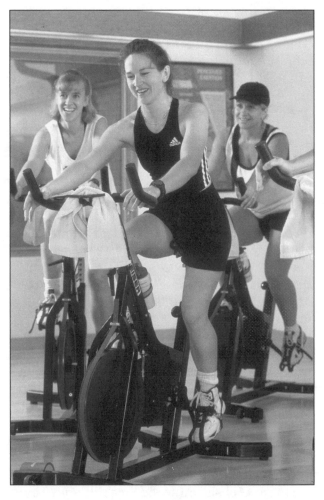

Find and maintain your "steady state," and get ready for vast improvements in your cardiovascular endurance.

are performing. You can use your heart rate as a tool to determine your intensity. Before we get into specifics, let's discuss some basic terminology.

Heart Rates

Once you determine your resting heart rate and training heart rate, it will be easy to discover if you are working out too hard or too lightly. Amazingly, after only a few months of training, you will probably be able to estimate your heart rate within a couple of beats. For example, during your warm-up, your heart rate may be around 100 beats per minute. But when you accelerate into a speed play drill, you will perceive that you are exerting more energy, and you are. Your training heart rate will correlate quite closely with how you feel.

Resting Heart Rate

This is your body's heart rate at rest, or your pulse rate taken approximately one hour before your normal waking time. Monitoring your resting heart rate (RHR) is one way to check for changes in your fitness and health levels. RHR is very much genetic. Pro tennis player Bjorn Borg had an RHR of 35 beats per minute. Borg was in fabulous shape, but so was Olympic track star Jim Ryan, whose RHR was 75 beats per minute.

Following are three ways to determine RHR:

1. Have someone gently wake you up and take your pulse one hour before your normal waking hour. Count the pulse for one whole minute.

2. In the evening, lie down in a supine position with some calming music and allow your body to relax without any distractions. Breathe comfortably for about 20 to 30 minutes. Count the pulse for one whole minute.

3. Wear a heart rate monitor to sleep and glance at it just as you are starting to wake. Record this number seven days in a row. Add them together and divide by seven. This will give you a true average of your RHR.

If you record this figure regularly and notice that your numbers are increasing by 10 percent, it means that you are overtraining or overstressed, or that your body is starting to break down or become ill. If this is happening, take the day off and pamper yourself by resting, getting a massage, or just training very lightly and easily for a couple of days until your RHR gets back to your normal average. On the flip side, if you notice your RHR dropping slightly, that is one indication that your cardiovascular fitness level is improving. When this happens, your heart has to beat fewer times each minute to sustain your normal body functions.

Power Point
Use your RHR to track changes in your health and fitness.

Maximum Heart Rate

This is the maximum recommended number of times your heart can contract in any given minute.

Following are three ways to determine maximum heart rate (MHR):

1. An easy, relatively accurate way to determine your MHR is by using this age-predicted formula: 220 – age = MHR (for men); 226 – age = MHR (for women).

2. In *The Heart Rate Monitor Book,* Sally Edwards suggests performing a long hill sprint or series of hill sprints after warming up. Give all-out, extreme effort until your heart rate reading no longer rises and you approach exhaustion. The final number is your MHR. Obviously, if you use this method, you should use a heart rate monitor and be supervised by a medical professional. This method is definitely not recommended for beginners or sedentary individuals.

3. A maximum stress test performed by a physician in a clinical setting requires you to walk on a treadmill while a doctor measures all of your vital signs. The walk turns into a jog and then a run. However, as the treadmill speeds up, so does the grade. Soon you can barely breathe as you are moving your feet as quickly as you can. Your doctor keeps asking if you are OK and you are supposed to nod yes as you push yourself to your limit. At the moment you reach your limit, you have achieved your MHR.

Recovery Heart Rate

This is the heart rate typically determined two minutes after the cardio portion of your workout is finished. Determine your recovery heart rate by counting your pulse for one minute. The only difference

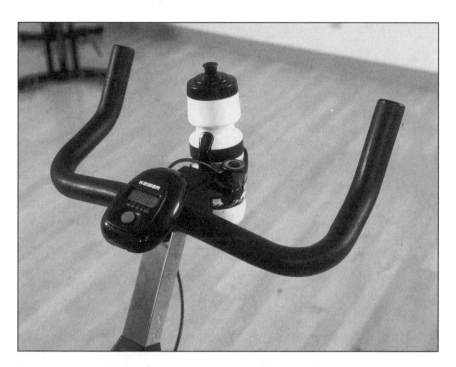

You can keep track of you heart rate with the Keiser bike's unique counter—all you need is a chest strap. The counter also gives you your speed, time, distance, and calories burned.

between recovery heart rate and RHR is that your recovery measure is taken after exercise. Record this number frequently since it is another method of determining cardiovascular fitness. The faster the number drops, the better. And the sooner it drops, the quicker you can perform another drill or interval on your bike.

Training Zones

In Power Pacing we concern ourselves with two training zones, the low training zone and the high training zone. When you know your training zones, you can increase or decrease your workload accordingly. For example, if your low training zone is 80 to 100 beats per minute and your actual heart rate at that low training zone is 120 beats per minute, you should decrease your intensity. If your high training zone is 140 to 170 beats per minute and your heart rate monitor shows that you are pedaling at 190 beats per minute, once again you should slow down and release some tension on the dial.

1. The low training zone is 50 to 70 percent of MHR.

Determine this zone by using this formula:

_____(MHR) × .50 = _____Low end figure

_____(MHR) × .70 = _____High end figure

Example for a 40-year-old man with an MHR of 180:

180 × .50 = 90

180 × .70 = 126

This person's low training zone is 90 to 126 beats per minute. He should allow his heart rate to drop to this level during the warm-up, between intervals, and during the cool-down. If his heart rate is higher than 126 beats per minute, he should perform a recovery, breathing, or mind/body meditation drill while flushing at a slow pace.

2. The high training zone is 70 to 90 percent of MHR.

Determine this zone by using this formula:

_____(MHR) × .70 = _____Low end figure

_____(MHR) × .90 = _____High end figure

Example for a 40-year-old man with an MHR of 180:

180 × .70 = 126

180 × .90 = 162

This person's high training zone is 126 to 162 beats per minute.

When beginners who have led sedentary lives start training, it is recommended that they stay in the low training zone for the first two weeks, taking part in two to three workouts per week for a maximum of 20 minutes. This allows for an easy break-in period that will help ward off excessive seat soreness. They may progress to the next level as they feel comfortable or as prescribed by their doctor or certified fitness professional.

If you have been regularly exercising a minimum of twice a week and lead an active lifestyle, it is recommended that you start out Power Pacing two to three times a week for a maximum of 30 to 40 minutes. Feel free to spend 60 to 80 percent of your workout in the high training zone. A good rule of thumb is if you perform two 4-minute songs or drills in the high training zone, then you should perform one song or drill in the low training zone to help recover.

If you have been regularly exercising three or more times a week quite vigorously for three or more months and lead an active lifestyle, you could Power Pace three or more times a week for 40 to 60 minutes. Because Power Pacing is such a high-intensity workout, remember to take a day off between workouts to do some other type of cross-training activity such as weight training. This provides your body and mind with a rest. And if you awaken to a faster than normal RHR, BE SURE to take a day off. You probably have been overtraining. Otherwise, feel free to spend 70 to 80 percent of your workout in the high training zone. Again, if you perform two (or three) 4-minute songs or drills in the high training zone, then you should also perform one song or drill in the low training zone to help recover.

Power Point
Your level of fitness will determine the length and intensity of your initial Power Pacing workouts. No matter what shape you're in, take a day off now and then so you don't burn out.

There is less perceived exertion for some people when pedaling a Power Pacer than when stepping up and down on benches or doing aerobics because there is no pounding to remind them that they are fatigued. Richard Cotton did a study with the American Council on Exercise (ACE) to determine the relationship of heart rates to intensity for group indoor cyclists. Cotton suggests that pressure to keep up with better-conditioned classmates and direction from instructors to keep the pace compounds the problem by pushing beginners beyond their physical abilities.

ACE's study looked at the heart rates of five subjects ages 23 to 35 during a 30-minute class. Their heart rates climaxed at 85 to 96 percent of their age-predicted MHRs and remained high for most of the workout. Conditioned athletes shouldn't work higher than 85 percent of their MHR according to ACE, and less fit exercisers should not exceed 65 to 75 percent. ACE suggests that high intensity levels may be acceptable for those who are fit, but intensity makes these classes overly demanding for beginners.

ACE makes the following recommendations:

1. Do some stationary cycling for a couple of weeks, interspersing high- and low-intensity work before joining a cycling class.

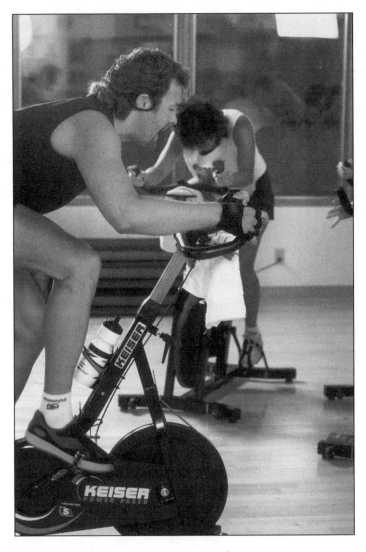

Avoid the pressure to keep up with your instructor. Go at your own pace.

2. Exercise at your own pace. Don't be intimidated by the high speeds and furious intensity of others around you. Slow your pace when necessary.

Modifying Intensity

One great and unique characteristic of Power Pacing is being able to modify your intensity. Intensity is evaluated as a measure of your heart rate, how your muscles feel, and how you feel in general. Do not compare your intensity to that of someone else. If someone else can do a standing climb with heavy resistance and you can only manage a seated climb with moderate resistance, that's fine. Your fitness level will increase, and soon you will be capable of a standing climb.

Following are four ways to modify intensity when Power Pacing:

1. Change body position: The first way to heighten or reduce intensity is to change your body position. For example, moving your body to the aggressive riding position from the basic or upright position forces the hamstrings into a lengthened state. Thus, moving from a shorter, more relaxed state, as in the basic position, to the aggressive position in which the hamstring muscles are contracted intensifies your workout. The aggressive position is also more difficult because the participant must have flexibility and torso strength in order to hold the position properly. Also, when standing, all of your body weight is put onto the pedals, which requires more muscle fibers to activate, thereby increasing the intensity. Play around with different body positions, and you'll quickly discover which ones really challenge your muscles!

2. Slow down or speed up: The second way to alter your intensity is to speed up or slow down your pedal speed. Adding more speed to your pedal stroke will increase the intensity of the drill. Always make sure you are in control if you are speeding up.

3. Add or decrease resistance: Changing resistance is another way to modify intensity, but it is not a constant variable. In other words, decreasing resistance doesn't always mean you will decrease intensity. For example, in a standing climb the use of medium resistance is going to provide a consistent comfort zone while performing at a comfortable cadence. If you decrease resistance when standing, you will have to speed up your pedal stroke, which increases intensity. If you add resistance beyond a medium level when sitting or standing, you will also increase your workload and intensity.

4. Use mindful focus and breathing drills: The fourth way to modify intensity is through mindful focus or breathing drills. When you focus your mind on an exciting thought, such as winning a race, you will stimulate your body into an arousal state that will help to slightly increase intensity. The breathing drill used for recovery in the basic drills section can be used to help decrease intensity when you focus on a long exhalation through the mouth and a quicker inhalation

Intensity of Drills and Positions

Body position	Hand position	Basic drill	Speed	Resistance
Seated upright	None	Seated upright	Slow	Light
Seated basic	Overhand	Flushing	Medium	None
Seated basic	Hook	Seated climb	Slow	Light
Seated basic	Hook	Seated climb	Medium	Medium
Seated basic	Hook	Fast hammer	Fast	Light
Vertical jog	Vertical jog	Vertical jog (moving)	Slow	Medium
Standing basic	Hook	Standing climb	Medium	Medium
Vertical jog	Vertical jog	Vertical jog (still)	Slow	Medium
Standing aggressive	Aggressive	Standing climb	Slow	Medium
Standing aggressive	Aggressive	Standing climb	Medium	Medium
Standing aggressive	Aggressive	Fast hammer	Fast	Light

through the nose. This type of relaxed breathing helps to calm the body down by delivering more oxygen to the working muscles.

If your goal is to reduce fat, some experts demand that you Power Pace within your target heart rate zone because aerobic exercise burns fat. However, other experts maintain that if you pedal at a higher intensity, your metabolic rate will increase, therefore burning more calories throughout the day. Our recommendation is that you

Heart Rate Diary and Pacing Log Chart

Day/Date	RHR	Pacing time	Low zone	High zone	2-min. recov. HR	Comments on wrkt
Sun 2/5	70	30 min.	15 min.	15 min.	120 BPM	It felt easy today.

do high-speed/resistance pedaling in addition to cycling within your training zone for the prescribed amount of times appropriate for your fitness level. Begin exercising in your low training zone for safety. You will be more likely to stick with your program. Later, as you learn to enjoy Power Pacing, add some speed work. You may be a budding cyclist or have the potential to be an Olympic-level athlete.

Use the heart rate diary and pacing log chart on page 61 to document your workouts. Over the course of your training, you may notice improvements in your Power Pacing workouts. For example, you may observe a quicker recovery period, slower RHR, and feelings of less perceived exertion for the same amount of work. This diary/log will help you keep track of the changes that indicate you are moving toward your goals.

Whether you are training for the Tour de France or just looking to improve your overall fitness, monitoring your intensity is a very important ingredient. A heart rate monitor can provide you real-time information concerning your training and performance. Or simply check your carotid pulse several times during your Power Pacing workout. Knowing your heart rate levels can help you prevent overtraining and give you a better chance of reaching your Power Pacing goals.

WARM-UP AND COOL-DOWN

In this chapter you will be learning how to prepare yourself properly for a vigorous Power Pacing workout while also learning the proper way to cool down, stretch, and recover at the end of each workout. References to warm-up and cool-down will appear in the chapters following this one. Each time you see them, you should refer back to this chapter.

Power Pacing Warm-Up

The warm-up is the first important part of your workout. This is the time when you get on your bike, set your goals, focus your mind on the work you are about to do, limber up your upper body, and get your legs ready for the more vigorous and demanding drills. The entire warm-up is done while riding. Think of warming up the body from head to toe as you are pedaling with light tension and a slow speed.

The following warm-up will prepare you to begin the more vigorous cycling drills. Take your time to understand effectively the skills involved. Each time you warm up in all of your Power Pacing workouts, refer back to this example.

Total time: 6 to 8 minutes

1. Start by taking a big, cleansing breath while bringing your arms up over your head. Then bring them back down while exhaling. Do this about four times. Next, reach for the sky

with your right arm and reach toward the floor behind you with your left arm, opening up and stretching out the muscles on the side of the rib cage area (figure 6.1). Repeat on the other side. Do each side twice.

2. Bring your arms down next to your body and begin limbering up your neck. Turn your head slowly from side to side bringing your chin over each shoulder.

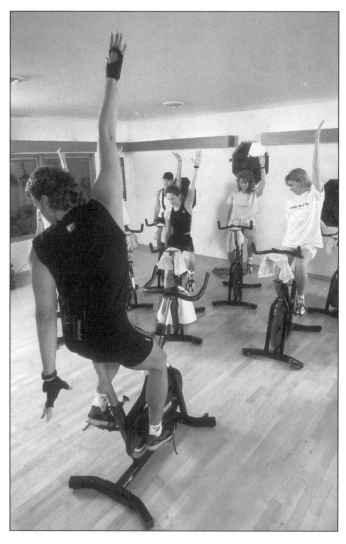

Figure 6.1 Always begin your workouts with a warm-up routine.

3. Now tilt the head from side to side bringing your ear toward each shoulder.

4. Next, tilt your head to the side and drop your chin down in front of you so you are looking at your navel. Then roll your head to the opposite side by making a half circle. Do not tilt your head back. Repeat this slow swinging motion a couple of times so that you stretch out the back of the neck and release the tension.

5. Lift your shoulders up toward your ears and press them back and down several times until you feel your neck muscles start to relax.

6. Roll your shoulders with big circles, moving forward, up, back, and down. Then reverse directions.

7. Rotate your shoulders forward without lifting them up and down. Now rotate them backward, squeezing your shoulder blades together.

8. Stretch both arms straight out in front of your chest, lace your fingers, and round your upper back, feeling the stretch through the upper shoulder blade area.

9. Lace your fingers behind you and stretch them up and back, feeling the stretch through the front of your shoulders and upper chest region. Keep your chest lifted the entire time, and do not bend forward. See figure 6.2.

10. Place your hands in an overhand grip, round your upper back, and tuck your hips under so that you feel a stretch throughout the whole spine. Your head should be down with your chin on your chest.

11. Keeping an overhand grip, move into a reversed basic riding position as you feel the opposition stretch opening up your chest and abdominals.

12. You should perform each movement and exercise a minimum of four times and hold the stretches for at least 10 seconds.

Power Point

Avoid fast, jerking motions, or ballistic stretching, as this may cause soreness and injury.

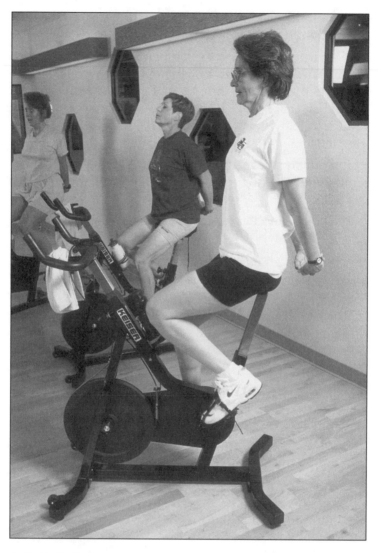

Figure 6.2 Power Pacing is a total body workout! Make sure you take the time to warm up your upper body.

13. Continue pedaling with light tension and a slow speed in a basic riding position. This point in the warm-up is a good time to check your alignment and technique. First, make sure your knees are tracking directly over your ankles. Refrain from allowing your knees to come inside the width of your feet or from bowing out. If this is happening, you may want to recheck your seat height. Next, look at your ankles. They

should be in a relaxed position without pointing your toes down or dropping your heels. It is also important to press through the center of the forefront of your feet. Take care not to ride on the outside or inside of your feet, as doing so will put additional stress on your knee joints. Last but not least, relax your toes inside your shoes. If your feet start to cramp during your workout, simply lift your toes up then relax them back down. This stretches not only your toes but the arches of your feet as well.

14. Continue riding at a slow to medium speed with light resistance for the remainder of your warm-up.

Cooling Down

The cool-down phase of your workout is always performed after the cycling component and should be the last thing you do. It is important to take the time to flush slowly to thoroughly recover the heart rate to the low end of your low training zone, which is about 50 to 60 percent of your MHR. Refer back to page 56 if you need to review the calculation. When we refer to a cool-down throughout this book, always refer back to the stretching drills explained later in this chapter.

Introduction to Stretching

A multitude of variables affect your flexibility. On warm days you are like a rubberband, while on cooler days you're tight. Yet regardless of the temperature or time of day, stretching is essential to good flexibility. The more flexible you are, the better cyclist you will be. Increased flexibility gives your muscles a longer range of movement, allowing for fuller extension and contraction. You can reach for a water bottle, and crouch into a lower aerodynamic position with ease.

Power Point
A millimeter of increased flexibility is as difficult to attain as a two-mile-per-hour increase in speed. Don't skip the stretches and let your body stiffen up!

Flexibility also determines coordination. Poor flexibility leads to poor posture, and in cycling good posture is a necessity. Your body is constantly changing positions, and good posture will help keep your body symmetrical and balanced, allowing you to perform your routine with control and grace. Flexibility helps you off the bike as well. A flexible joint and muscle requires less energy to move. You will feel less stiff as you age because of increased blood and nutrient supply to joint structures. And with better flexibility, you will be less likely to injure your low back, shoulders, and knees in your daily routine.

Strength and flexibility are the keys to enduring those on-the-bike postures that would otherwise make your back unhappy. Bend forward from your waist while on the saddle of your Power Pacer. At about 15 degrees of flexion your back muscles (erector spinae) eccentrically lengthen. These muscles are holding you in position. Your erector spinae muscles are constantly contracted during Power Pacing. When you bend a little further, to about 45 degrees, your hips engage. Bend past 90 degrees and your back is supported by ligaments. Pain receptors called nociceptors are in these ligaments. That's why, whenever you bend beyond 15 degrees, it's important to place your hands on the handlebars to support your back.

Stretching is paramount to preventing injury. If an area of your body is inflexible, another part must compensate. When your hamstrings are tight, your quadriceps must contract harder to overcome that tension. When that happens, you're more likely to injure the overworked quadriceps muscle. Likewise, a lack of flexibility in the hip flexors and hamstrings may be a prime cause for on-the-bike back pain. This is because your back muscles are overcompensating for your weaknesses. To avoid overcompensation, stretch the agonist and antagonist of each major muscle group you use for Power Pacing. The antagonists to your triceps are your biceps. The antagonists to your quadriceps are your hamstrings.

Other benefits of stretching include the following:

- Stretching alleviates delayed onset muscle soreness because it relaxes potential muscle spasms.
- Stretching the quadriceps, hamstrings, and hips helps protect the knees and lower spine from injury, as sudden movements will be less likely to cause muscle strains or tears.
- Stretching helps prevent neck pain and decreases the debilitating effects of carpal tunnel syndrome.

If you're running low on time and think you can afford to skip stretching, think again. The increase in flexibility and coordination, as well as injury prevention, are paramount to cycling success. If stretching is neglected, the consequences will likely catch up to you fast.

Stretching Drills

Each of the following upper and lower body stretches should be performed after you have recovered your heart rate as mentioned earlier. A slow, continuous stretch is desired. Hold each stretch for a minimum of 20 seconds to fully relax the muscle. Slowly stretch to the limits of joint motion until you feel tension in your muscle, then relax. Go for comfort.

Soft music in the background is nice. Stretch without a teeth-clenching, red-ballooned face and monitor your joints, muscles, and tendons. Your body will adapt to the stretching positions, and soon you will stretch comfortably.

Power Point

Always fully engage the tension lever on the bike so the pedals don't move when cooling down and stretching.

Upper Body Stretches

The following upper body stretches are done on the bike:

1. Stretch your low back (quadratus laborum, erector spinae) by performing the reversed basic riding position. Use your arms for support, lift your chest, and keep your abdomen in.

2. Stretch your upper back (latissimus dorsi) by performing an opposition stretch. Grab the left side of your handlebar with your hands a few inches apart. Stabilize your body with your left hand and pull with your right hand to stretch the right side of your torso (see figure 6.3). Switch hands and repeat.

3. Lower your chin to your chest and tuck your hips under, rounding your back.

4. Press yourself into an upright position and pull your shoulder blades back (scapular retraction) to stretch your chest.

5. Interlace your fingers and reach overhead and backward for a chest and shoulder stretch.

6. As in the beginning of the warm-up, reach one arm up and the other back down behind you in opposition. Turn your head and focus down at the floor where you are reaching. Repeat on the other side.

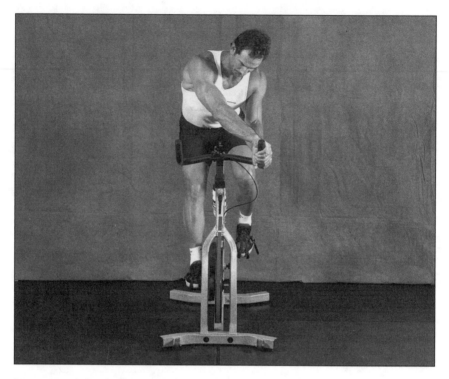

Figure 6.3 Upper back (latissimus dorsi) stretch.

7. Remain upright and grasp your right elbow with your left hand up behind your head and pull it up and back, stretching your triceps and latissimus dorsi. Switch arms and repeat.

8. Interlace your fingers low behind your back and feel the front of your shoulders and chest stretch out. Keep lifting your chest while you stretch.

9. Interlace your fingers behind your head, elbows out. Lift your chin and chest and open your elbows even more to stretch the front deltoids and chest area muscles.

10. Place one hand over the top of your head covering one ear with your palm and gently stretch out the side of your neck. Repeat on the other side.

Power Point
Exhale as you move into each stretch.

On-the-Bike Lower Body Stretches

The following lower body stretches are done on the bike. They are not recommended if you have problems with balance or are not very flexible. A definition of not very flexible would be if you have a difficult time sitting up straight on the floor and touching your toes while your legs are straight out in front of you. If you fit into this category, try the variations in the next section for standing on the floor or skip these stretches and do the floor stretches on page 76.

1. After you have fully engaged the tension lever, remove your left leg from the pedal and place it on the handlebar. Grip the handlebar on either side of your leg and lean forward for a hamstring stretch. Pull your toes back with your right hand for an additional calf stretch. Or, if you can't reach, use a towel to help by placing it over the forefoot and holding it on each end. Push through your heel as your toe pulls back and work with as straight a leg as possible (see figure 6.4).

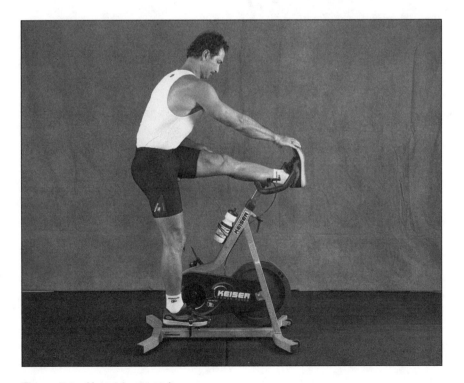

Figure 6.4 Hamstring stretch.

2. Sit upright for a spinal twist with your right leg extended on the handlebar. Rotate your torso to the right, keeping the spine upright and the hips square to the front of the handlebar. Push through the arch of your right foot as you twist. Feel your spine getting longer with each inhalation and twist further with each exhalation.

3. Rest the outside of your right ankle on the left overhand grip position of the handlebars so your knee is bent and pointing to the right in a figure four position. Move your hips slightly to the left so you are sitting on the middle of your right buttock. Inhale as you lift your chest and exhale as you lean your chest forward toward your knee, stretching your hip (gluteus and piriformis), as shown in figure 6.5.

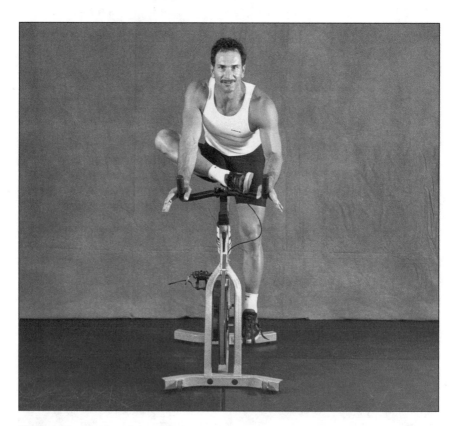

Figure 6.5 Hip stretch.

4. Center yourself back on the saddle and carefully remove your foot from the handlebars. Bend your right knee and grasp the top of your right ankle or foot with your right hand. Press your knee back as you lift your chest (see figure 6.6). It is not necessary to press your foot hard into your hips. This stretch will be felt in the front of the hip and in the quadriceps, or front of the thigh. If you feel any pressure in your knee, release your ankle. For more stability feel free to lean forward and place your left hand in an overhand grip.

5. Repeat all of the above stretches on the opposite side in the same order.

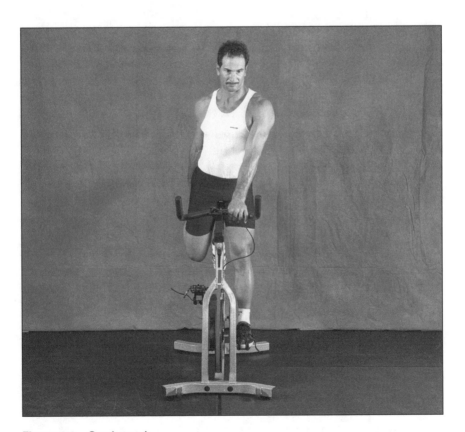

Figure 6.6 Quad stretch.

Posture and Stretching Do's and Don'ts:

1. Do contract your abdominal muscles.
2. Don't arch your back too much; keep a neutral spine.
3. Don't let your head pull your neck too far forward.
4. Do adjust your handlebars so you can sit upright.
5. Do perform deep long stretches only after the cycling workout is finished and you have performed a recovery drill to bring your heart rate down.
6. Don't hold your breath.
7. Do breathe from your diaphragm.
8. Don't bring your foot up on the handlebar if you lack balance or flexibility.
9. Do relax and breathe deeply into each stretch for at least 20 seconds during the cool-down.

Off-the-Bike Lower Body Stretches

These lower body stretches are done off of the bike. They are more appropriate for the person who is not very flexible in the hamstrings and low back.

1. Stand facing the side of the bike and bring your left heel up on the center frame of the bike. Place one hand on the handlebar and the other on the seat as you bend forward from the hips, stretching out the hamstring (see figure 6.7).

2. While holding onto the bike, cross your left ankle on top of your right thigh and bend your supporting (right) leg as you allow your hips to slide back as if you were squatting. Make sure the knee and toes of your support leg are both facing the bike, as shown in figure 6.8. Take care not to pull on the bike, as it may tip.

3. Standing upright, take hold of your left ankle or foot behind you as you bend your knee to stretch out the front of your thigh and hip. Make sure to tuck your hips under and don't press your heel to your buttocks too firmly.

4. Bring your right foot close to the bike and lunge the left foot back with a straight leg until you feel a stretch in the front of

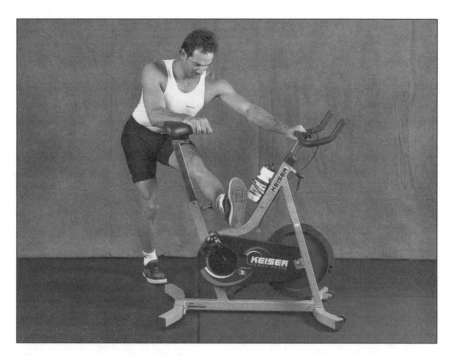

Figure 6.7 Hamstring stretch.

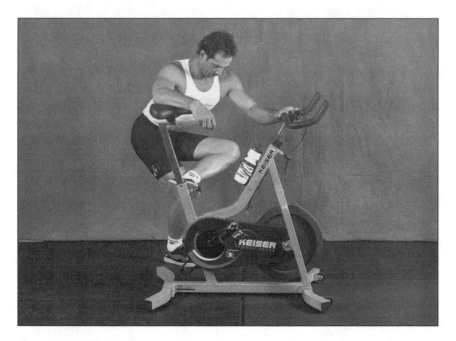

Figure 6.8 Hip stretch.

your hip and in the calf muscle of your left leg. Press your left heel toward the floor.

5. Repeat all of the above stretches on the opposite side in the same order.

Additional Stretches

These stretches are done on the floor. They would be appropriate for people who have difficulty with balance or flexibility. They are also appropriate for anyone to do after finishing the on- and/or off-the-bike stretches. If you happen to be short on time, it's okay to skip these stretches, as long as you've performed all of the previous upperbody and one of the lower body routines.

1. Lie on your back with your legs straight and draw your right knee into your chest. Hold onto the back of your thigh, not the top of your knee. Push through your left heel, drawing your left toes back. Feel the stretch on the top of your left hip and in the back of your right buttocks area. Try to keep your tailbone on the floor.

2. Slowly twist your right knee across your body toward the floor on the opposite side. Your left hand should be on the outside of your right thigh helping you twist. Turn your head to the right and press the back of your right shoulder into the floor. Feel the opposition stretch in the spine and outside of the right hip.

3. Bend your left knee, keeping the sole of the foot on the floor. Next, place the outside of your right ankle on top of your left thigh close to your left knee. Draw your legs in toward your chest as you hold onto the back of your left thigh. Your right hand should be between both legs, and your left hand should be on the outside of your left leg. Feel the stretch deeper on the outside of your right hip.

4. Repeat 1, 2, and 3 on the other side.

5. Sit on the floor with your back against a wall and the soles of your feet together. Hold onto your ankles. Keep your back upright and press your knees toward the floor. Feel this stretch in the inner thigh and groin area.

6. For a deeper stretch stay in the same position as 5, lean forward, and use your elbows to press your knees further down to stretch out your inner thighs.

7. Sit upright against the wall while you cross your legs comfortably. Place the backs of your hands on your knees. Close your eyes and focus on your breathing. Inhale counting to 2, then exhale counting to 4. Allow your body to settle and relax.

Close your eyes and breathe deeply from your diaphragm. With each exhalation relax every muscle in your body. Consider how Power Pacing has allowed you to undergo a profound change. Your body achieved a peak experience, and now you are drifting back to reality—but before you do, relish those moments of perfection. Feel your legs churning so fast that even you cannot believe your speed. Experience a powerful sense of self. See your body as strong and supple. In the next few moments, let these suggestions reinforce themselves, then slowly come out of your relaxed state. As you do, you can program yourself to feel any way you want to.

Prepare yourself for high-intensity Race and Pace, covered in chapter 7. Understand that you can modify your intensity as you wish. You may achieve a oneness of mind, body, and breathing that cannot be equalled.

RACE
AND PACE

Race and Pace is a variety of timed high-intensity drills combined with periods of recovery. It strengthens your muscles, fortifies your heart and lungs, and increases your ability to sprint on your bike. Race and Pace will teach you to recruit more muscle fibers for your workout. At first, you may try to pedal fast, but your muscles may not respond. Pedaling fast is a skill that improves with practice. It is a neurological mind/body training effect. Soon, with diligent training and athletic drill practice, your speed and power increase.

After you have warmed up, try this simple test: pedal as fast as you can for 30 seconds. Count your revolutions per minute (rpms). This is done by counting the number of times your right foot makes one complete revolution in one minute. After one month of twice weekly interval training and athletic drills, test yourself again. You should not be surprised to see a 10-percent increase in your performance.

Interval Training

Years ago, fitness enthusiasts were instructed to increase exercise intensity gradually until they reached a steady state. Steady state referred to a target heart rate zone just below anaerobic threshold. Their goal was to endure this level of intensity for as long as possible. Recently, however, research has shown that it is better to vary the intensity of a workout. Rather than mindlessly pounding the pavement or covering a certain distance at a steady pace, athletes are now encouraged to use interval training.

Interval training involves changing your intensity throughout your workout, alternating high-intensity speed training and low-intensity recovery. While continuous, slow distance training increases aerobic capacity only, interval training improves both aerobic and anaerobic capacity.

Power Point

For best results, intersperse steady, aerobic Power Pacing with more intense bouts of training.

Short, frequent periods of training are more beneficial than longer programs for certain populations; some folks are simply incapable of maintaining a longer routine. Beginners, the very deconditioned, and those with certain medical conditions—such as asthma—should start with several condensed sessions and progressively make them longer and more frequent.

To begin, make pedaling intervals equal in intensity to your normal steady state program. Follow this with a rest/recovery segment performed at a reduced workload. A workout may last for only 15 minutes with 5-second intervals and 15-second rest periods. Gradually, the Power Pacing workout will double and so will the pedaling intervals, while the rest periods remain the same.

As your conditioning improves, increase the intensity of your workouts. Interval training will improve your aerobic capacity, or your body's ability to deliver oxygen to your Power Pacing muscles. $\dot{V}O_2$max represents the greatest amount of oxygen your body can take in and use to provide energy to your muscles during your best cycling effort. In other words, it is the rate your quadriceps, hamstrings, gluteals, and calf muscles efficiently use nutrients from oxygen.

The faster your body can deliver oxygen to your cycling muscles, the higher your $\dot{V}O_2$max will be. You can improve your $\dot{V}O_2$max by about 20 percent, but the remainder of it is contingent upon genetics. World-class cyclists are genetically gifted with a high $\dot{V}O_2$max, but they, too, need interval training to increase it and give themselves an edge. Improving your $\dot{V}O_2$max depends on how you tolerate lactic acid buildup. Lactic acid is the by-product of your muscle metabolism that causes a burning sensation as you exceed your anaerobic threshold. Interval training increases your ability to tolerate lactic acid buildup and therefore enhances your $\dot{V}O_2$max.

Power Pacing Intervals

Interval training drills burn fat and build endurance, speed, and recovery. Shorter workouts make intervals a pleasant diversion from

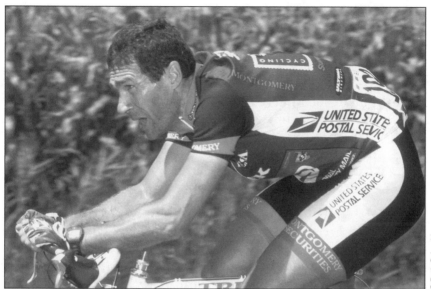

Even world class cyclists need interval training to put them at peak performance.

© Beth Schneider

your long, slow distance training. The faster, more intense velocity and the challenging body positions may be exhilarating, yet uncomfortable at first as your heart rate and breathing skyrocket and your thighs feel rubbery—but soon intervals will energize you!

Power Pacing intervals teach your muscles to use stored energy so you can endure several sprints with short recovery periods. During the first 10 seconds of a fast hammer, you rely on your adenosine triphosphate-creatine phosphate (ATP-PC) cycle, or your quick energy system. Fast hammers, therefore, require your muscle cells to adapt to speeds required for sprinting. From 10 to 90 seconds, your lactic acid system provides energy to complete your pedaling.

Speed play is interval training without a system. You decide how hard to work and you control your intensity based on your tolerance. Speed play is more creative than timed intervals, and it's a great change of pace from a prescribed program. Just let loose and progress to your anaerobic threshold and beyond! Be sure to recover appropriately.

Level 1 Cyclists

Level 1 cyclists can pedal an outdoor bicycle at about 10 miles per hour on a flat grade without wind. They are generally new to physical training and are considered novices in Power Pacing.

An aerobic interval Power Pacing program for the level 1 cyclist is low intensity. The work and rest intervals occur only at an intensity within your aerobic system. The work period is performed at an intensity that's just a bit higher than your steady state. (Steady state is comfortable pedaling, with slightly labored breathing.) The recovery period, however, is somewhat lower in intensity than your steady state.

The time in each interval ranges anywhere from 15 seconds to three minutes, coinciding with the length of each tune. If you do not relish watching the clock, simply accelerate toward the finale of each song. Then flush until the next tune begins. Add a one-minute interval each week to your training until you are sprinting a dozen one-minute cycles. Power Pace a maximum of three times per week.

Level 2 Cyclists

Level 2 cyclists can pedal their outdoor cycles on level ground, with no wind, an average of 12 to 15 miles per hour. They are somewhat athletic and generally have been physically active for several years.

Climb on your Power Pacer and warm up with six to eight minutes of comfortable pedaling, as described in chapter 6. Increase your pace, but not too fast. Pedal at 70 percent of your maximum for one minute until you begin huffing and puffing. If your legs burn, you are pedaling too fast. Slow down a bit in order to stay below your anaerobic threshold and to prevent deadening lactic acid from permeating your muscles. You cross your anaerobic threshold when your legs ache and you can hardly catch your breath. If you remain aerobic, but very close to your lactic acid/anaerobic threshold, you will last longer.

Remain at this upper limit for one minute. Take a one-minute, easy-pedaling intermission. Pedal another minute interval. This is an equal time speed burst. Continue to alternate one-minute, upper-limit pedaling with one minute of easy pedaling. Equal time speed bursts allow you to train at the upper limits of your aerobic capacity, thereby increasing your ability to tolerate lactic acid and increasing your anaerobic threshold.

Recovery intervals allow lactic acid to circulate so you are primed for your next effort. Lactic acid is converted into glucose by your liver and muscle cells to energize the remainder of your workout. Easy pedaling is the best way to disperse lactic acid; it is even more effective than stretching or massage.

Another 30-second speed burst program consists of the following: after your warm-up, fast hammer at 65 percent of your maximum speed for 30 seconds. Flush at 70 percent of your MHR for 30 seconds. Any 30-second speed burst uses energy from your lactic acid system.

Fast hammers require 30 seconds of explosive action followed by periods of active recovery flushing.

Level 3 Cyclists

Level 3 cyclists can average between 18 and 20 miles per hour on level roads with no wind. They are very athletic and may enjoy Power Pacing to enhance their competitive cycling performance. For level 3 Power Pacers, increase the speed or resistance during your intervals. Power intervals train your heart muscle more effectively than a single bout of continuous training. During power interval training, your heart must overcome a greater resistance. This leads to improved heart rate function. Your heart empties more completely, increasing your stroke volume and cardiac output. Your brain experiences a huge sense of appreciation when the interval is complete.

A level 3 interval training program is very high in intensity as rated on the perceived exertion scale. The perceived exertion scale, or Borg scale, is a subjective rating of your intensity from 6 (very low) to 20 (very high). A 6 on the scale correlates to 60 beats per minute, and a 20 would feel like you are at an MHR of 200 beats per minute. You can last up to 15 seconds at a perceived exertion of 18 during a level 3 cycling program. A rating of 18 would therefore be considered very difficult and should be followed by a recovery interval. Use this approach only if you are highly fit and athletic.

Fast hammer at 95 percent intensity for 15 seconds. Then take a 45-second flushing break to get ready for the next bout. Because your work/rest cycle is relatively short, you can repeat the cycle 10 to 20 times within a Power Pacing workout. Create your own level 3 interval training program by alternating work and rest intervals. First, pedal at a high intensity for a short duration. The work interval is performed for 15 seconds or less at a level greater than your anaerobic threshold. Your rest interval occurs in your aerobic system and is considered active recovery. This allows for the removal of lactic acid from your working muscles.

A level 3 program on the opposite end of the anaerobic spectrum recommends you increase your resistance to simulate a moderate hill climb. After your initial warm-up, described in chapter 6, ride hard for 30 minutes as if climbing a 10-mile hill. Back off and flush for a five-minute period before doing the complete cool-down you learned earlier. Perform this routine only twice a week. Be sure your body has recovered between training sessions. Consider this the ultimate form of cross-training, providing a specific benefit to your outdoor cycling performance.

To mirror small hill climbs, begin with a six- to eight-minute warm-up. Then do three 30-second work intervals with a one-minute rest between each set. Pedal with a smooth, easy, steady state cadence for 10 minutes mimicking a long, flat road. Then do three more intervals. As this becomes easier, increase your intervals to one minute. This helps to increase your aerobic power and will help you match the same scenario during your outdoor performance.

Power Pacing and Your Metabolism

Power Pacing increases your metabolism. During fast hammers, your body preferentially burns carbohydrates rather than fat, but intervals allow you to perform more work, increasing your exercise post-oxygen consumption (EPOC). While your feet are propped comfortably on the La-Z-Boy, your fat stores release energy to replace depleted carbohydrates. EPOC, the "afterburn," is the total number of calories you burned long after you completed your workout. This total number depends on the amount of work performed, regardless of whether it was continuous or intermittent.

Your metabolism remains elevated up to 15 hours after an interval training session. One investigation cited in the February 1995 issue of *Prevention* magazine examined a group of cyclists who trained moderately four times a week, burning 400 calories per session. Another group trained moderately twice a week, but on the other two days performed interval training. The intervals only burned 250 calories per session, but two days of moderate exercise combined with two days of intervals incinerated nine times more fat than four days of moderate exercise. Because of the afterburn effect, there was a greater increase in EPOC for the interval group. Therefore, interval training on your Power Pacer burns more total fat and calories than continuous training.

Athletic Drills

Athletic drills are very similar to the drills a road cyclist uses when training. Each one is based on intervals of some sort or examples of what you may encounter on a real road ride, such as big hills, rolling hills, a race, or maybe just a relaxing ride. Each of these drills are made up of the basic drills you already read about in chapter 3. They are combined with athletic drills to form a program called Race and Pace.

Power Point

As you perform each of these drills, imagine yourself outside on a real bike. Try using the music examples to help motivate you during your ride.

SPEED PLAY TRAINING

The speed play training drill is performed by randomly performing the basic drills. Depending on your fitness level, select basic drills and frequently change the time you spend doing them, your body and hand positions, the speed, and/or the resistance.

Imagine yourself riding outside in a particular location and select music that will help you visualize your environment. An example may be to imagine yourself riding through the hills and valleys of the Irish countryside while you play some upbeat Celtic music. Or imagine yourself in control of a spaceship racing around dodging asteroids and Darth Vader's death ray as you play the theme song to *Star Wars*.

Speed Play Training Drill

Body position	Hand position	Basic drill	Speed	Resistance	Time
Seated basic	Overhand	Fast hammer	Fast	Medium	15 sec.
Seated basic	Overhand	Seated climb	Medium	Medium	30 sec.
Standing aggressive	Aggressive	Standing climb	Slow	Medium	20 sec.
Seated basic	Overhand	Flushing	Slow	None	30 sec.
Vertical jog	Vertical jog	Vertical jog (still)	Slow	Medium	15 sec.
Standing basic	Hook	Standing climb	Slow	Heavy	10 sec.

Repeat these twice for a four-minute song.

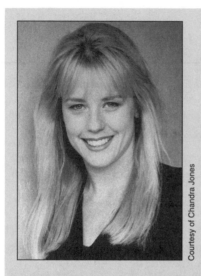

Courtesy of Chandra Jones

Chandra Jones's Athletic Drill Workout

My favorite interval training drill is the pyramid climb because of the great results it gives me. Since I often work as a stuntwoman, I am asked to repeat a difficult stunt over and over for the camera crew until they can get the right shot. This requires a lot of quick-burst energy or anaerobic power, often with short rest periods in between each take. Interval training is perfect to keep me in shape for stunt work!

I like to do a Pyramid Climb variation in which I only pyramid up, making each working interval a bit more challenging as I go. Before I train with this drill, I warm up with about 15 minutes of basic seated drills.

The soundtrack for the movie *Mortal Combat Annihilation* is perfect for this drill. Many of the songs on that soundtrack have hardcore, driving rhythms that I find great for motivation.

After warming up, begin easy with 10 seconds of a fast hammer in the seated basic riding position. Eventually work your way up to 50 seconds of fast hammer in an aggressive standing position, always recovering 10 seconds in between. After that, recover by flushing for three minutes and repeat the whole sequence two more times, finishing up with a proper cool-down.

Chandra has been an international workshop presenter and instructor for more than 10 years. She works as a personal trainer to many celebrities, as well as a stuntwoman/actress and fitness model. She has been featured in numerous fitness videos, television shows, and publications, such as *Ms. Fitness* and *Oxygen*.

EQUAL TIME SPEED BURSTS

Pick a certain amount of time, such as 15 or 30 seconds, and perform a basic drill at a high intensity level. Then use the same amount of time with a different basic drill at a low intensity level. Try the sample program shown in the table. Select music that is very upbeat and fast, such as "Heartbreaker" by Pat Benatar or "Go Daddy Go" by Big Bad Voodoo Daddy, to help keep you moving during the challenging intervals. During the recovery phase, make sure to breathe deeply.

Equal Time Speed Bursts Drill

Body position	Hand position	Basic drill	Speed	Resistance	Time
Seated basic	Hook	Fast hammer	Fast	Light	30 sec.
Seated basic	Overhand	Flushing	Medium	None	30 sec.
Standing aggressive	Aggressive	Standing climb	Medium	Heavy	30 sec.
Seated basic	Hook	Seated climb	Medium	Medium	30 sec.
Seated basic	Hook	Seated climb	Medium	Medium	30 sec.
Seated basic	Overhand	Flushing	Slow	Light	30 sec.

Repeat these twice for a six-minute song.

PYRAMID CLIMB

The pyramid climb drill is designed to teach your body how to sustain longer, more challenging work intervals along with fixed periods of rest. This drill has two unique qualities:

Pyramid Climb Drill

Body position	Hand position	Basic drill	Speed	Resistance	Time
Seated basic	Hook	Fast hammer	Fast	Light	30 sec.
Seated upright	None	Flushing	Slow	None	30 sec.
Seated basic	Hook	Fast hammer	Fast	Medium	60 sec.
Seated upright	None	Flushing	Slow	None	30 sec.
Standing basic	Cupping	Standing climb	Medium	Medium	90 sec.
Seated basic	Cupping	Seated climb	Medium	Medium	30 sec.
Standing aggressive	Aggressive	Standing climb	Medium	Medium	120 sec.
Seated basic	Overhand	Flushing	Slow	None	30 sec.
Standing aggressive	Aggressive	Standing climb	Medium	Medium	90 sec.
Vertical jog	Vertical jog	Vertical jog (still)	Slow	Medium	30 sec.
Seated aggressive	Aggressive	Fast hammer	Fast	Light	60 sec.
Seated basic	Hook	Flushing	Slow	None	30 sec.
Seated basic	Overhand	Fast hammer	Fast	Light	30 sec.
Seated upright	None	Flushing	Slow	None	30 sec.

Total duration is 11.5 minutes.

1. The first work interval sets the timing for all of the recovery periods. If you choose 30 seconds for your first work interval, all of the subsequent recovery periods will be 30 seconds long.

2. The first work interval also sets the amount of time you add to or subtract from the other work intervals. Therefore, using the example in 1, your next work interval would be 60 seconds, then 90 seconds, and so on. When you're ready to come down the pyramid, you subtract 30 seconds from the last work interval. The music you use for the pyramid climb should be very upbeat and driving, just like the music you selected for the speed bursts drill. Once again, make sure to focus on lengthening your exhalations during the recovery phases.

HILL SPRINTS

Hill sprints simulate riding over rolling hills and include three equal time interval working phases. The table below offers a sample hill sprint routine using 20-second intervals. The first interval is performed seated, simulating climbing the first part of the hill. The second interval is performed standing, simulating climbing the second part of the hill or the steepest part. Finally, the third part, the downhill phase, is performed seated while executing a quick-paced drill such as a fast hammer.

Hill Sprints Drill

Body position	Hand position	Basic drill	Speed	Resistance	Time
Seated basic	Overhand	Seated climb	Slow	Medium	20 sec.
Standing basic	Hook	Standing climb	Medium	Medium	20 sec.
Seated aggressive	Aggressive	Fast hammer	Fast	Light	20 sec.

Repeat these four times for a four-minute song.

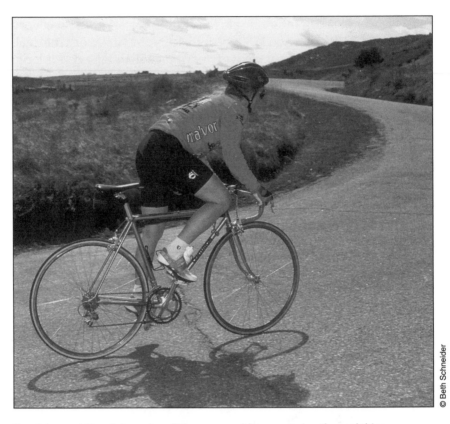

© Beth Schneider

Practice your hill sprints and you'll have no problem mastering the real thing.

There are no recovery periods in this drill so it is very important to incorporate a breathing drill, such as inhaling for two counts and exhaling for four counts, during the first part of each hill climb to help calm the body down slightly. Quick, upbeat music, as in the last two drills, is great for this drill as well.

LONG HILL SPRINTS

Long hill sprints are performed by standing and climbing for the whole song, either using a considerable amount of tension and climbing slowly or reducing the tension slightly and pedaling a little faster. Changing your body position is another way to vary the intensity of this drill.

Long Hill Sprints Drill

Body position	Hand position	Basic drill	Speed	Resistance	Time
Standing basic	Hook	Standing climb	Slow	Medium	20 sec.
Standing basic	Hook	Fast hammer	Fast	Medium	20 sec.
Standing aggressive	Aggressive	Standing climb	Medium	Medium	20 sec.
Vertical jog (still)	Vertical jog	Vertical jog (still)	Slow	Medium	20 sec.
Vertical jog (moving)	Vertical jog	Vertical jog (moving)	Slow	Medium	20 sec.
Standing aggressive	Aggressive	Fast hammer	Fast	Light	20 sec.

Repeat these twice for a four-minute song.

Conquering Hills

Try the following techniques and you'll breeze right through those long hill sprint routines!

Sensory Awareness Method

One of Kris's favorite techniques to maintain motivation during this drill is what he calls "the sensory awareness method." Find a song you like that is going to help you get motivated to climb a long hill and dub in messages or short lines of visualizations to help keep you motivated. It's like having your mind speak to you out loud, providing you with positive thoughts. First, select a location and music that is going to give you the feeling of being there. Then dub in short descriptions every 10 to 15 seconds that relate to your senses of sight, smell, taste, touch, and hearing.

Example: Location—Climbing a big hill in Hawaii

Music: Sounds of steel drums, crashing water, and birds

You're starting to climb the hill. See the ocean to your left and the rich tropical foliage to your right.

Hear the crashing of the waves against the shore.

Lick your lips and taste the salty air.

Smell the exotic fragrance of magnolia and jasmine in the air.

Feel the warm wind at your back helping to get you up the hill.

See a big macaw flying out ahead of you with a five-foot wing span. Watch his tail feathers as they float in the wind. Match your pedal stroke with the same smooth, flowing feeling.

It's morning; see the orange glow over the top of the hill. You are halfway there.

Hear the loud sound of the macaw as he leads you up to his nest where he has something you've wanted for a very long time.

Feel the cool humidity and moisture in the air as you ride under a row of large palm trees.

You've finally made it to the top. Park your bike and jump in the nest to find your gift.

Goal Setting With Silence

Another simple method Kris created is "goal setting with silence." This also works very well for a long hill sprint drill. Decide on a goal to focus your mind on, close your eyes, and think about that goal as if it is already happening. Notice the feeling of excitement and arousal this strong thought process allows. Select music that has lyrics in it describing getting higher, reaching, climbing, or getting to the top. This can be a very powerful way to meditate for success as you are working out. "Dreams" by Van Halen, "Reach" by Gloria Estefan, and "Feet Don't Fail Me Now" by Phil Collins are all very good songs for this drill.

RACE SIMULATION

Race simulation is similar to the speed play drill on page 85 except that you visualize being in a cycling race. Here's an example: the starting gun is about to go off. You stretch your torso into a reversed basic riding position one last time. Pow. Get moving; fast hammer. Assume your seated aggressive riding position and make a break for it. Shift into a heavy gear allowing you to stand in the aggressive riding position. Hold that position as you power away from the pack. You are way ahead, so you sit upright and take a drink. Cruise comfortably in your seated basic riding position holding your lead. Fast country rock music, such as "The Devil Went Down to Georgia" by the Charlie Daniels Band, is fun for this drill.

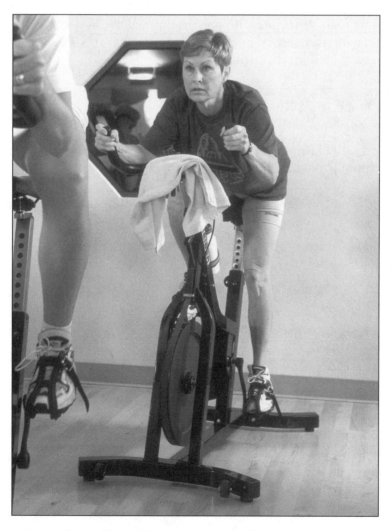

Get into your racing position and hammer toward the finish line!

RECOVERY DRILL

The recovery drill focuses on calming and cooling the body after vigorous, more challenging work has been performed. You may use relaxation techniques, a breathing drill (such as inhaling for two counts and exhaling for four counts), or simply decrease the intensity of your workout by incorporating the flushing and seated upright basic drills. The object is to relax your body by decreasing the speed and resistance of each drill while closing your mind to all thoughts and distractions. Direct your focus inward to calm down the body and heart rate. Associate with your body and let it relax. Slow ballads, calming instrumentals, or new age music that has flowing water work very well for this drill.

Recovery Drill

Body position	Hand position	Basic drill	Speed	Resistance	Time
Seated basic	Overhand	Flushing	Slow	None	30 sec.
Seated upright	None	Seated upright	Slow	Light	30 sec.
Seated upright	None	Breathing drill*	Slow	Light	30 sec.
Seated basic	Overhand	Flushing	Slow	None	30 sec.

Repeat these twice for a four-minute song.

*Inhale 2 counts and exhale 4 counts.

Race and Pace Workouts

Now that you have a good understanding of the basic and athletic drills and how to modify the intensity of each, it is time to create your first few actual workouts. Race and Pace is a workout training program consisting mostly of basic and athletic drills. Following are three examples of Race and Pace workouts. Select music that is going to motivate you to finish each drill. Have fun!

In each of these workout examples the warm-up and cool-down should be taken from chapter 6. Refer back to chapter 5 if you are not sure whether your heart rate should be in the low or high training zone.

Twenty-Minute Start-Up Race and Pace Workout

Song	Drill	Time	HR zone
1	Warm-up	4 min.	Low
2	Warm-up	4 min.	Low
3	Speed bursts	3 min.	High
4	Hill sprints	3 min.	High
5	Speed play	3 min.	Low
6	Cool-down	3 min.	Low

Feel free to extend your cool-down if you need more time to recover.

This is a start-up program that only lasts 20 minutes—great for the level 1 cyclist.

Forty-Minute Intermediate Race and Pace Workout

Song	Drill	Time	HR zone
1	Warm-up	4 min.	Low
2	Warm-up	4 min.	Low
3	Hill sprints	4 min.	High
4	Long hill sprints	4 min.	High
5	Speed play	4 min.	Low
6	Pyramid climb	12 min.	High
7	Race simulation	4 min.	High
8	Cool-down	4 min.	Low

This is an intermediate-level workout and would be great for the level 2 cyclist.

Sixty-Minute Intermediate-Advanced Race and Pace Workout

Song	Drill	Time	HR zone
1	Warm-up	4 min.	Low
2	Warm-up	4 min.	Low
3	Speed bursts	4 min.	High
4	Long hill sprints	4 min.	High
5	Speed play	4 min.	Low
6	Pyramid climb	12 min.	High
7	Recovery drill	4 min.	Low
8	Hill sprints	4 min.	Low
9	Speed bursts	8 min.	High
10	Long hill sprints	4 min.	High
11	Recovery drill	3 min.	Low
12	Cool-down	5 min.	Low

This is an intermediate- to advanced-level workout great for the level 2 cyclist who is looking for a challenge or the level 3 cycling participant.

Race and Pace drills simulate actually racing on your outdoor bike. You can also use Race and Pace drills to enhance your outdoor performance. You might pretend you are in a lead pack being chased. Or you can use speed bursts to increase your aerobic power. Competitive outdoor cyclists find that Race and Pace drills are very valuable cross-training tools for enhancing their racing performance.

Race and Pace athletic drills can help you build your speed and power whether you are a level 1, 2, or 3 cyclist. Always begin with a warm-up and finish with a cool-down. Progress gradually, week to week, and slowly begin to lengthen your work intervals and shorten your rest periods. If you are a road racer, use imagery to visualize breaks, sprints, and hill climbs. Although Race and Pace workouts do not require music, a hard, driving beat may increase arousal and performance.

RHYTHMIC DRILLS

No other indoor cycling program simulates the precision and detail involved in cycling like Power Pacing rhythmic drills. You'll learn how to perform moves a mountain biker uses when making sharp turns, pedaling up and down steep hills, dodging tree limbs, and more! The drills in this chapter can be performed slowly to practice proper riding technique, core stability, balance, and coordination and/or combined with different variations of tempos and rhythms to create routines for more advanced training.

Rhythmic drills are energizing! You'll learn how to perform your new moves to the beat of your favorite music. Time passes quickly. Before you know it, you have completed an entire song using a rhythmic drill. Even the least musical folks can follow the beat of a rhythmic drill.

At first, follow the directions for each drill without worrying about the music so that you master the proper techniques. Once you have mastered them, enjoy pedaling to the beat. Soon you will be combining rhythmic drills, working every muscle in your body to the beat of your favorite tunes.

Pedaling to the Beat

As a general rule, the faster a rhythmic drill is performed, the more advanced it becomes. If you are just starting out and have never done these movements before, perform them slowly with control and focus mainly on your form, technique, and correct body positioning on and off the seat.

Music selection for rhythmic training drills is very specific. The beats per minute of your music should be close to 125. You can determine this by counting how many downbeats you hear in a song for 30 seconds and multiplying it by two. A downbeat is the song's main, accented beat and is usually the beat you'd tap your toe to. Most club music is this tempo because it is easy to dance to. The CD *Ultimate Dance Party '97* has many great songs on it that work very well for rhythmic training and can be purchased at most music and discount department stores.

If you use music that is the prescribed tempo, many of these drills can be performed at three different speeds: slow, medium, and fast.

- The slow speed is performed by counting two downbeats as each individual leg completes a downstroke. This is very similar to the speed of a slow hill climb or muscle recruitment drill.

- The medium speed is performed by matching each individual leg or downstroke to the downbeat of the music. This would be similar to a quicker hill climb or having a feeling of marching to the beat of the music.

- The fast speed is performed by moving your downstrokes double time to the beat of the music or, in other words, twice as fast as the medium speed. This may be similar to a fast hammer tempo.

Power Point

Unlike the speed, which varies, the resistance for rhythmic training drills is always medium whether standing or seated. Remember, before you stand up you must always add a little more resistance because in the standing position your perception of resistance will be lighter due to the weight of your body on the pedals.

Power Pacing's 10 Rhythmic Drills

Let's get started learning the 10 rhythmic drills. Take your time practicing them to a slow tempo first and then try them a bit faster. Often you will be asked to change your lead leg to emphasize the opposite leg. If you notice that you have a hard time slowing down, add a bit more tension so you always remain in control of your pedal stroke. You should never feel as if the bike is pushing you.

POWER LEG/FLOAT LEG

The power leg/float leg drill is performed in a seated position. Your goal is to focus on one leg (the power leg) while the other (the float leg) just moves along for the ride. Although your float leg should not be doing any of the work, make sure you still keep both feet in the pedals while riding (figure 8.1).

As you are performing this drill, focus on the full circle of the pedal stroke—down, back, up, and forward—taking time to recruit all of the muscle groups in your power leg. This is the same movement that you learned to do slowly in the basic muscle recruitment drill. This is a great drill to perform in your warm-up in order to work each isolated leg equally.

Leg speed: slow, medium, or fast

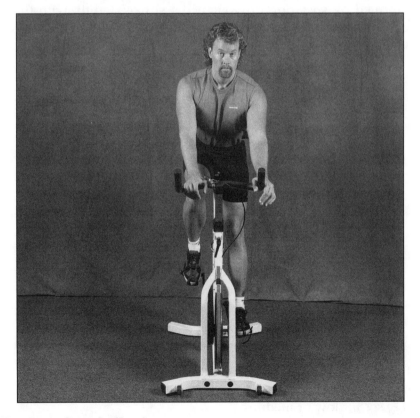

Figure 8.1   Power leg/float leg.

LEAD LEG

This drill is very similar to the power leg/float leg drill, which focuses on one leg. However, because you're in the standing position, you must use the float leg slightly in order to turn the pedal stroke around.

This drill strengthens each individual lead leg, but in a standing position. It is great for mountain biking when you need to make a sharp turn going uphill, requiring you to press heavily with the inside leg as you turn your front wheel to the side.

Leg speed: slow or medium

ROLL AND SWITCH

This drill is used as a transition to change power or lead legs. It is performed by speeding up your pedal stroke slightly with three individual downstrokes and then starting into the former speed with the opposite leg leading.

This movement is typically performed with power leg/float leg or lead leg drills. It can be done in the standing or seated position. You may want to try it also as a transition between seated and standing variations.

The following are ways to use roll and switch:

1. Perform power leg/float leg leading with the right leg, roll and switch sitting, then start power leg/float leg leading with the left leg.

2. Perform power leg/float leg leading with the right leg, roll and switch standing, then sit down and start power leg/float leg leading with the left leg.

3. Perform lead leg with the right leg, roll and switch sitting, then stand up and start lead leg with the left leg.

4. Perform lead leg with the right leg, roll and switch standing, then remain standing and start lead leg with the left leg.

Roll and switch allows you to gain control of your pedal stroke when slowing down or speeding up, without coasting, in order to change the lead leg.

Leg speed: slow or medium

DOWNSTROKING AND UPSTROKING

These actions simulate the basic drill variations of muscle recruitment for the quads and hamstrings, except they are done with less resistance so you can pedal to the rhythm of the music you select.

Downstroking focuses on pushing the bottom of your feet toward the floor. Upstroking focuses on wiping your feet on the floor without pointing your toe. Do not pull up on the cage. Power leg/ float leg can be used as a transition between upstroking and downstroking. Try the following exercises:

1. Perform eight power legs with the right foot (again, that is the number of times your right foot completes one revolution). Perform 16 downstrokes alternating legs for 16 counts. Start counting with the right foot. Perform eight counts of power legs leading with the left foot, then 16 upstrokes alternating legs starting with the right foot for 16 counts. Remember that upstrokes are counted by how many times the leg curls up into the upstroke to engage your hamstrings.

2. Perform the same combination using a ratio of four to eight.

3. Perform the same combination using a ratio of two to four.

Leg speed: slow, medium, or fast

LEAN OVER LEG

Lean over leg is performed by slightly moving your upper body toward the downstroking leg just as mountain bikers do when they are leaning into a turn or going up a hill (see figure 8.2). One difference is that a regular mountain or road bike would be doing the side-to-side motion, while on a stationary bike you're the one that moves.

This drill can be performed seated or standing. When standing it is very important not to lean very far. If you feel any movement of the bike, you know you are leaning too far. Just move slightly side to side to the rhythm of the music.

Keep your hips over the seat with your knees over your feet. Do not let them move side to side. The movement should involve only a slight lateral flexion of the spine.

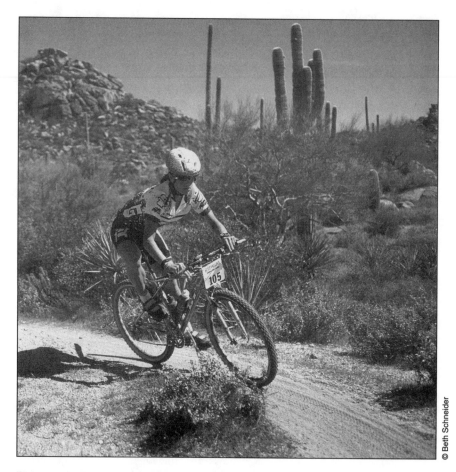

© Beth Schneider

Figure 8.2 This mountain biker uses lean over leg to follow the curve.

Your handgrip should remain relaxed and your weight should never be on the handlebars. The hook grip works best for this drill unless you are in an aggressive body position, in which case you would use the aggressive grip.

Leg speed: slow or medium

DIPS

Standing in a basic riding position with your hands in a parallel grip, allow your elbows to bend to the side and float your chest up and down. Make sure to keep the weight on your legs, not on your arms. Allow your hips to shift back so that your spine remains neutral (see figure 8.3). Do not round your back as you go down.

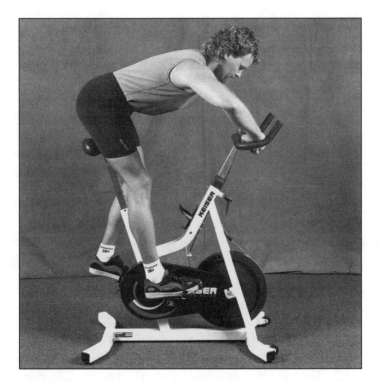

Figure 8.3   Dips.

When you perform dips in the seated position, your hands should be in the seated parallel grip.

Because this is an upper body horizontal motion (the chest lowers while the hips move back), it is possible to have the upper body moving at a different tempo from the legs.

Try the following combinations:

1. With the leg speed slow, allow your upper body to dip down as your right leg moves into the downstroke and up as your left leg moves into the downstroke.

2. With the leg speed slow, allow your upper body to dip down with each downstroke and up with each upstroke.

3. With the leg speed medium, allow your upper body to dip down as your right leg moves into the downstroke and up as your left leg moves into the downstroke.

4. When performing a standing dip, try adding a roll and switch in a vertical jog body position to change lead legs, and then dip down with the opposite lead leg.

5. Try combining lean over leg movements with dips. Perform lean over leg 16 times. (You would count each time you move to one side as one. Moving right, left, right, left would be considered four times.) Then dip eight times. Dips are counted by the number of times you go down. For more of a challenge, try a ratio of eight lean over legs to four dips or four lean over legs to two dips.

6. Perform the lean over leg eight times, dip three times, then roll and switch to change lead legs. Now do the whole combination again, but lean to the opposite side to start.

Leg speed: slow or medium

DIGS

Digs are performed standing in a basic or aggressive riding position with the hands in a hook grip or aggressive grip. Your whole body is moved forward and back, maintaining a neutral spine with your head at the same level (see figure 8.4). In other words, when you perform the forward motion, do not drop your upper body down toward the handlebars. Because this is a front-to-back motion, it is possible to have the upper body moving at a different tempo from the legs.

A variation of the dig can be performed on a diagonal when the body is moving forward at the same tempo as one single lead leg is downstroking.

The backward motion of the dig imitates the movement a mountain biker makes to get up a hill faster and more efficiently. Likewise, mountain bikers use the forward motion of the dig to get down a hill more quickly.

Here are some different dig combinations to sharpen your mountain biking skills:

1. With the pedal speed slow, the dig can be performed at a slow tempo moving forward for two downbeats and back for two downbeats.

2. With the pedal speed slow, the dig can be performed at a medium tempo moving forward and back to the beat of the music.

3. With the pedal speed medium, the dig can be performed at a fast tempo moving forward and back double time to the beat of the music, which is quite fast.

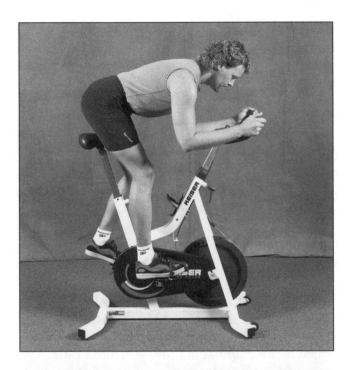

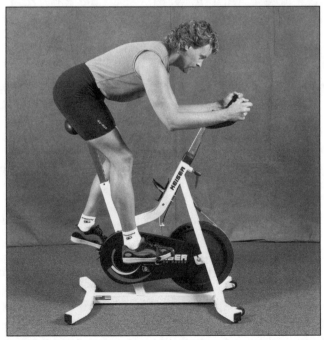

Figure 8.4 Digs.

4. With the pedal speed medium, the dig can be performed with a rhythm change—move the body forward one downbeat, back one downbeat, and then hold forward for two downbeats. Then do the opposite by moving back one downbeat, forward one downbeat, and back holding for two.

5. With the pedal speed slow, match the forward motion with the downstroking of the right leg. Place the hands in a diagonal grip with the right hand forward in the hook grip. As you dig forward, move the torso slightly on a diagonal toward the right front. Then as the left foot downstrokes, move the upper body back slightly to the left rear diagonal.

6. Repeat example 5 three to seven times front and back. Then, perform one roll and switch in a vertical jog body position and you are ready to do a diagonal dig in the opposite direction.

7. Digs can also be combined with lean over legs and dips. For example, with a medium speed in the legs, lean over leg eight times total, dip down and up four times (remember, dips are counted by the number of times you move down), and dig as in example 4 twice (forward, back, hold forward, back, forward, hold back). This would be a total of 32 downbeats.

Leg speed: slow or medium

SLIDES

Slides are very challenging and are performed only in the aggressive riding position. They emphasize maintaining a neutral spine when standing. Slides strengthen the low back muscles, allowing you to stand for longer periods in an aerodynamic, or aggressive, position without losing control.

Start in an aggressive seated position with your hands in an aggressive grip. Next, lift your hips up and back about one to three inches, lengthening the spine into a standing aggressive riding position (see figure 8.5). In the correct standing position, the low back acquires a natural lumbar curve and the hamstrings feel lengthened.

If, during the three sample exercises, the muscles on top of your thighs become fatigued, you are probably rounding your back and tucking your hips under. Never lift your chest or put weight on your forearms.

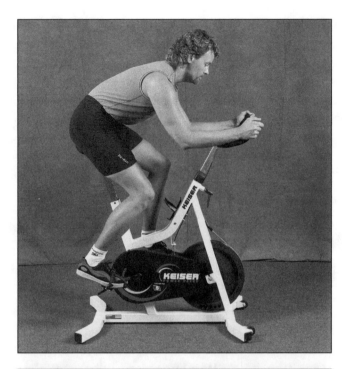

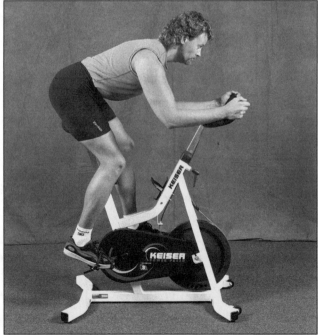

Figure 8.5 Slides.

1. With the pedal speed slow, medium, or fast, slide your hips up and back eight, four, or two counts up and eight, four, or two counts down.

2. With the pedal speed slow, medium, or fast, slide your hips up and back for a count of one and down for a count of three.

3. Combine slides with the lean over leg drill in the aggressive riding position. Perform lean over leg seven times, sitting down on the eighth count, and then perform slides up and back for a count of two and down for a count of two.

Leg speed: slow, medium, or fast

SEATED PUSH-UPS

Cyclists of all types need to have strong upper bodies to control their bikes, especially in the dirt and gravel. These two seated push-up

Seated Push-Ups Drill

Body position	Hand position	# of reps
Seated basic	Overhand	8
Seated basic	Corner	8
Seated basic	Overhand	4
Seated basic	Corner	4
Seated basic	Overhand	2
Seated basic	Corner	2
Seated basic	Overhand	1
Seated basic	Corner	1
Seated basic	Overhand	3
Seated basic	Corner	1
Seated basic	Overhand	2
Seated basic	Corner	2
Seated basic	Overhand	1 (hold 2 cts.)
Seated basic	Corner	1 (hold 2 cts.)

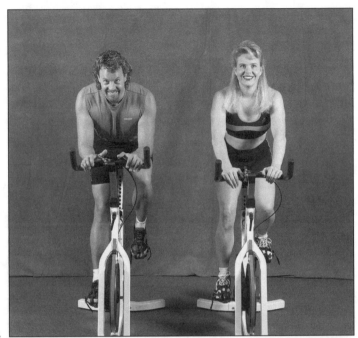

A

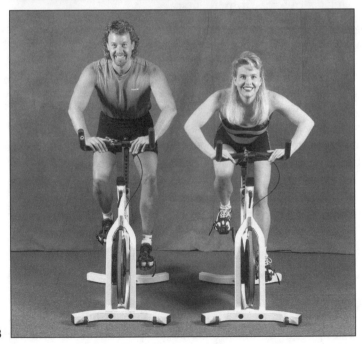

B

Figure 8.6   Seated push-ups *(a)* isolating the triceps and *(b)* focusing on the chest and shoulders.

variations will help you accomplish this by isolating the triceps and chest muscles (see figure 8.6).

To isolate the triceps, start in the overhand grip and press your body weight into the handlebars, allowing the elbows to move straight down parallel with the wrists.

To focus more on the chest and front of the shoulders, start in the corner grip and press your body weight into the handlebars, allowing the elbows to move out slightly.

Try out these combinations to work your upper body:

1. Focus on the downward motion of each exercise to emphasize the eccentric contraction of the muscle being isolated.

2. Focus on pushing upward to emphasize the concentric, or shortening, contraction of the muscle being isolated.

3. Bend your arms slowly, focusing on both the downward and upward movements.

4. Perform different rhythmic patterns. For example, try the sample drill on page 108.

Leg speed: slow, medium, or fast

DIAGONAL GRIP AND SWITCH

Perform the diagonal grip and switch by moving from one diagonal grip to the opposite diagonal grip. To maintain balance and control, always move one hand and grip before switching the other hand. Never change both hands at the same time.

You can change your grip when doing a roll and switch seated or standing. Always have the same hand forward as the leg you are emphasizing.

This can also be used as a fun transition in an arm push-up combination. Try turning your head away from the hand in the hook grip.

Leg speed: slow, medium, or fast

Choreographic Styles

Choreographic styles are simple ways to combine rhythmic drills during songs. Following are choreographic methods and styles to help as guides. Each method should be used to format two or more rhythmic drills into a single four-minute song.

Diagonal Grip-and-Switch Combination Drill

Body position	Hand position	# of reps
Seated basic	Overhand	3
Seated basic	Corner	1
Seated basic	Overhand	2
Seated basic	Corner	2
Seated basic	Overhand	1
Seated basic	Corner	1
Seated basic	Overhand	1
Seated basic	Corner	1
Seated basic	Grip and switch	2

Freestyle Technique

With freestyle technique you start with a basic movement and add or subtract another movement, rhythm, or variation to make your workout more interesting. You can go from one rhythmic drill to another, playing with the speed and switching hand and body positions. The combinations are endless! This technique is great for beginners because they get to experience all the movements without having to remember what comes next.

As you move through each of these drills, take your time so that you really focus on the proper form and skill of each movement. There is no set time period or specific number of downbeats to stay within. Just focus all of your energy on proper riding technique.

Try the following routine:

1. Start pedaling at a medium speed and perform seated push-ups using an overhand grip.

2. Move to a diagonal grip with the right hand forward and focus on power leg/float leg with the right leg leading.

3. Roll and switch, and grip and switch, focusing on the opposite leg.

4. Increase tension a bit and focus on downstroking.
5. Next, with a slow tempo, perform lean over leg seated.
6. Slowly stand up and continue lean over leg with a slow tempo.
7. Change hand positions to a parallel grip and try some slow dips.
8. Move the hands to the hook grip, increase speed to a medium tempo, and lean over leg to the same tempo.
9. Change to the aggressive body position and continue lean over leg.
10. Sit down, slow down, and focus on upstroking in the basic riding position.

Count Down/Up Method

The count down method starts out with two different rhythmic drill movements performed 16 times, then 8, then 4, then 2. The count up method is just the opposite.

The following sample combination uses both variations of the seated push-up. Try it emphasizing the downward, or eccentric, accent one time and then the upward, or concentric, accent another time.

Perform 16 seated push-ups using an overhand grip and 16 seated push-ups using a corner grip. Then, 8, 8; 4, 4; 2, 2; and 1, 1. Now go the opposite way for the count up method.

Chorus/Verse Method

Many songs are made up of chorus and verse sections. The chorus sections are the same words or rhythmic phrases repeated over and over between the verses. To use this method you would select two different rhythmic drills and alternate them with the chorus and verse sections of the song. Just choose a song and two different drills and you're ready to go!

Try the following routine with the song of your choice:

Perform a lean over leg standing in a basic riding position during the chorus and seated push-ups using a corner grip during the verses. Repeat this until the song is over. It is a good idea to do a standing drill on the chorus and seated drill on the verse for variety and to work more muscles.

> **Power Point**
> Perform your drills with music of your choice. This improves the frequency, intensity, and duration of your Power Pacing.

Choreographic Build

Take three or four different movements and/or rhythms and piece them together. This is very advanced and should not be performed unless you have become comfortable with the movements and can perform each of them with perfect form. Never sacrifice form for speed.

The following sample choreographic build uses the lean over leg, dips, digs, and roll and switch:

With a medium tempo in the legs, combine lean over leg standing in a basic riding position eight times starting to the right side and counting each side as one. Follow this with two dips, moving down with the right leg and then four double dips moving down with each leg. Next, dig to the front four times total and then perform three diagonal digs to the right, change to a vertical jog body position, and perform one roll and switch. Now start the whole combination from the left.

Rhythmic drills can be as easy or as complex as you wish. Use the freestyle technique first and take the time to focus on your form. Once you feel you've mastered that, move on and try a choreographic build, which will challenge your mind as you have to remember the order of your combination patterns. Remember, rhythmic drills should always be done with medium resistance, and each one should start with a slow tempo and progress according to how confident you feel with the movements.

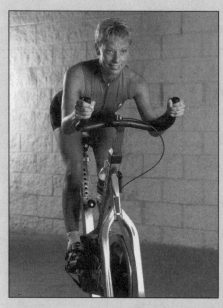

Tracy Schotanus's Rhythmic Drill Workout

Having been an aerobic dance champion, I enjoy movement with an emphasis on staying to the beat. Rhythmic training allows me to express that passion. My favorite rhythmic drills are the lead leg drill, lean over leg, and digs. The combination of these three rhythmic drills allows for many variations. One of my favorite songs, "Come on Ride the Train," works well for the following variations.

After completing a thorough warm-up as described in chapter 6 and four minutes of seated drills, it's time to stand up and play!

1. With medium resistance on the dial, stand up in a basic riding position and start to feel the rhythm and beat of the music.

2. Next, perform a lean over leg drill, moving left for two beats then right for two beats.

3. Now it's time to pick up the pace, so move to a medium speed. Be sure to keep your weight off of the handlebars and your abs held in for lower back support.

4. Slow it back down and change from a hook grip to a diagonal grip with the right hand forward.

5. Now focus on the right leg by doing a lead leg drill.

6. Next, move into a dig going forward as the right leg downstrokes and back as the left leg downstrokes.

7. After doing several forward digs, change to a diagonal and do a diagonal dig to the right.

8. Put 6 and 7 together by doing two forward digs and two diagonal digs to the right. Do this four times.

9. Change the pattern again with one forward dig and three diagonal digs to the right, then do singles to the front and side.

10. Slow it down a bit so you can roll and switch and repeat 5 through 10 on the left side.

After you've completed that, do the following choreographic build to a medium rhythm:

11. Do four lean over legs in an aggressive riding position. Start with the right side, counting each side movement as one beat.

12. Next, do one forward dig, three diagonal digs to the right, then another forward dig.

13. Quickly move into a vertical jog position and roll and switch so you can repeat 11 and 12, leaning left first.

Tracy is a seven-time Canadian National Aerobics Champion and World Silver Medalist. She has 15 years of experience in the fitness industry as a certified trainer, program designer, and international presenter and speaker. Tracy is also president and founder of Health Technologies Incorporated, a private personal health club in Calgary.

POWER PACING WORKOUTS

Everything you've learned so far is finally coming together—the basic drills, the athletic drills, and the rhythmic drills. Most important, you're learning how to combine and modify each one to suit your current fitness needs. Combined, these drills constitute Power Pacing and are the foundations of the workouts you are about to experience. Each of the following programs will give you the foundation for creating your own program.

We suggest that you start out with the 25-minute program if you are just beginning. As you feel more fit in a couple of weeks, challenge yourself by moving up to the 40- or 60-minute routines. Take your time, be patient, and most important, monitor yourself throughout the workouts not only by your heart rate but also by keeping a good eye on your form, making sure you are executing the drills properly and not going too fast without proper control. The resistance is up to you. Always use enough tension so you are in control of your pedal stroke. Pick out your favorite tunes and ride!

In the following programs a warm-up and cool-down are always referenced. Go back to chapter 6 if you need to review the components. If you have extra time after completing the warm-up components, just ride out the rest of the song with an easy pace, focusing on your form and control of your pedal stroke. You'll also notice that each drill is referenced by a page number so you can go back quickly and find an example to follow.

Whether you are seated or standing for each drill is up to you. If you feel you need to increase your heart rate, you may want to try standing up for the drill. You can always refer to chapter 5, which describes how to make cycling drills more or less challenging.

Your hand and body positions are up to you as well. Refer to chapter 2 if you need some ideas. Always remember to use the aggressive grip in the aggressive body position. The hook grip is the most common grip and is always a good position to stay in if you are unsure. Dips always use the parallel grip. Other than that, play and have fun changing as you go.

For every drill we recommend a heart rate zone, either low or high. See chapter 5 to determine what your low and high zones are.

Power Point

Once you have decided the order of each of your drills, select music and make yourself a tape to work out to. Make sure to put at least five to eight seconds of silence between songs when recording your music so you won't forget to take a drink of water after every song.

Twenty-Five-Minute Start-Up Program

This program should be the first Power Pacing workout you try after you have a good understanding of body positions and the basic drills. Since it is a beginning level and includes a low heart rate zone, you'll probably stay seated and remain in a basic riding position most of the time.

Forty-Minute Program

After you have practiced the start-up program two to three times for two weeks in a row, it's time to move on to a new challenge: the 40-minute program. During the drills that require you to be training in the high zone, try standing up more and getting into the aggressive body position. This will challenge you a bit more. During your long pyramid climb drills be patient and take it one interval at a time. If you start to feel at all lightheaded, back off a bit because you may be pushing yourself too hard. Remember, Rome wasn't built in a day. If you want the body of a Greek god or goddess, it's going to take some time.

Twenty-Five-Minute Start-Up Power Pacing Program

Song	Drill	Time	HR zone	Page #
1	Warm-up	4 min.	Low	63-67
2	Power leg/float leg	4 min.	Low	99
3	Speed bursts	3 min.	High	87
4	Seated push-ups	3 min.	Low	108-110
5	Lean over leg/ digs	3 min.	Low	101-102/ 104-106
6	Flushing	2 min.	Low	34
7	Cool-down	6 min.	Low	67-77

Forty-Minute Power Pacing Workout

Song	Drill	Time	HR zone	Page #
1	Warm-up	4 min.	Low	63-67
2	Warm-up	4 min.	Low	63-67
3	Hill sprints	4 min.	High	89-90
4	Lean over leg/dips	4 min.	High	101-102/ 102-104
5	Muscle recruitment	4 min.	Low	34
6	Pyramid climb	11.5 min.	High	87-89
7	Seated push-ups	3 min.	Low	108-110
8	Cool-down	5.5 min.	Low	67-77

Sixty-Minute Program

When you've been consistently riding and practicing for at least two months, it's time to take the 60-minute challenge. Train hard in the high zone drills and remember to put the same amount of effort into focusing on the recovery in the low zones. This peaking and recovering is what makes Power Pacing a very effective and challenging program. Are you ready? Take the challenge!

Mix and match these workouts and have fun with them. If you are unclear how to modify the intensity of each exercise, refer back to chapter 5, pages 58-62.

Sixty-Minute Power Pacing Workout

Song	Drill	Time	HR zone	Page #
1	Warm-up	4 min.	Low	63-67
2	Speed bursts	4 min.	Low	87
3	Long hill sprints	4 min.	High	90-91
4	Slides/digs	4 min.	High	106-108/ 104-106
5	Recovery drill	4 min.	Low	94
6	Pyramid climb	11.5 min.	High	87-89
7	Lean over leg/ dips	4 min.	Low	101-102/ 102-104
8	Hill sprints	4 min.	High	89-90
9	Lead leg	4 min.	High	100
10	Long hill sprints	4 min.	High	90-91
11	Seated push-ups	3 min.	Low	108-110
12	Recovery drill	3 min.	Low	94
13	Cool-down	6.5 min.	Low	67-77

Jill Watkins's Power Pacing Workout

As director of a YMCA, I get people of all shapes, sizes, and fitness levels in my classes. Power Pacing allows me to teach to all these different students at the same time. They simply vary their intensity to match their level of fitness by adding or subtracting tension, standing up or sitting down, or changing their body position.

The workout I am going to describe for you is great for someone who has just finished up two weeks of 20-minute start up workouts and is ready for the next step into a full 40-minute program.

Remember, if it says standing climb, you can always make it easier by sitting down. If you forget how to modify the intensity of one of the drills, check out chapter 5 for a quick review.

Song	Drill	Time	HR zone	Page #
1	Warm-up	4 min.	Low	63-67
2	Speed bursts	4 min.	High	87
3	Muscle recruitment	4 min.	Low	34
4	Lean over leg/dips	4 min.	High	101-102/ 102-104
5	Hill Sprints	4 min.	Low	89-90
6	Pyramid climb	4 min.	High	87-89
7	Digs and diagonal digs	4 min.	Low	104-106
8	Race simulation	4 min.	High	92-93
9	Seated push-ups	4 min.	Low	108-110
10	Cool-down	4 min.	Low	67-77

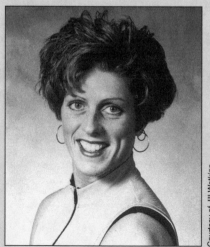

Courtesy of Jill Watkins

Jill is an Amateur Athletic Union (AAU) 1995 National/World Silver Medalist and 1996 Bronze Medalist in Double Step. She has been involved in fitness and management for more than a decade and currently holds the position of fitness director for the Worcester YMCA in Massachusetts.

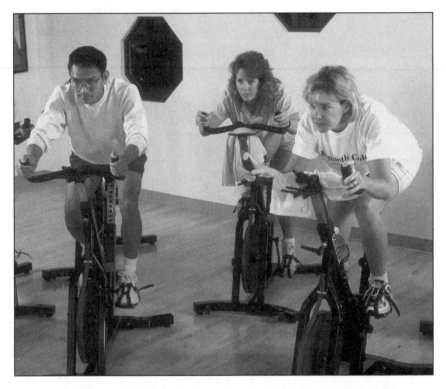

Once you've mastered the other programs, it's time for the 60-minute challenge!

You have now experienced Power Pacing at its best—the challenge of athletic training drills and the precise and flowing movements of the rhythmic training drills all in one powerful workout. The seated push-up drills should have made your upper body a bit stronger. Get ready for chapter 10. The cycling workout is the same as Power Pacing with one more element added to the end of the workout to make it more complete—strength training. So read on and get ready to pump up!

PACE AND SHAPE

Strength training must be an integral part of any exercise program in order to achieve total body health and fitness. You can dramatically improve the way you look, feel, and perform just by lifting weights. Pace and Shape—a program designed to work the upper body using free weights—as well as the Kris Kory Bike Band explained in chapter 11 allow you to reap the benefits of strength training without even getting off your bike! First you'll learn what you can look forward to with Pace and Shape. Then we'll show you how to put together your own Pace and Shape programs that you can easily add to your Power Pacing workouts.

What to Expect From Pace and Shape

Pace and Shape improves your outward appearance and has far-reaching effects on your physical well-being. You'll be able to sculpt your body, improve your health, and enhance your performance. When you add Pace and Shape to your Power Pacing workouts, you'll improve your cardiovascular fitness, muscular strength and endurance, body composition, and flexibility. Pace and Shape is your secret weapon for total fitness!

A Well-Sculpted Body

You no doubt desire a nice shape to your body. There is no better way to contour and streamline your physique than strength training. Although you cannot spot-lose body fat, you can tone up and increase the size of your muscles. This is the key to a firm, strong, shapely body. You can even use the upper body exercises in Pace and Shape to increase the size of your shoulders and upper back to create the illusion of a small waistline.

Because body type plays a major role in your development, you may derive different results from those of your buddy on the same Pace and Shape program. You may not want to grow slabs of muscle like a professional bodybuilder, but you can develop whatever muscle you have. Regardless of your body type, unless you inject illegal supplements, you should not be concerned about transforming into the Hulk.

There are three different body types:

• Mesomorphic—A mesomorphic body type is one with well-defined muscles on the trunk and limbs. These folks are broader in the shoulders and hips and narrower at the waist. They have a high muscle-to-fat ratio and look fit even without Pace and Shape. Mesomorphs who Pace and Shape notice a dramatic increase in strength and muscle mass.

• Endomorphic—An endomorphic body type is rounder, softer, and pear shaped with more fat surrounding the gluteals and thighs. Endomorphs' muscles are not well defined and they have a higher fat-to-muscle ratio. Power Pacing helps with fat loss, but they must be patient. Pace and Shape programs for endomorphs should focus on upper body development to balance their larger hip proportions.

• Ectomorphic—An ectomorphic body type is long and rectangular, flat chested, and slender in the hips, with no defined waist. Ectomorphs have poor muscle development with relatively low body weight. Folks with this body type have difficulty retaining muscle. Ectomorphs must be sure to take in enough calories to balance their Power Pacing caloric expenditure.

No matter which body type you possess, you will harvest the rewards of Pace and Shape—a leaner and stronger body. You'll see the improvement in your outward appearance, but more important, you'll also feel the difference.

Improvement in Your Health

The American College of Sports Medicine (ACSM) recommends that strength training be an integral part of an adult fitness program. This is because strength training not only produces cosmetic benefits but also delivers results you can feel as well as see. You can look forward to the following improvements in your health:

- Lower blood pressure
- Increase in food transit time through the colon to combat some types of cancer
- Increased bone density, thereby decreasing your chance for osteoporosis
- Increase in good HDL cholesterol
- More muscle helps prevent type II diabetes because additional muscle uses more oxygen and takes up extra sugar. Lower blood sugar levels are important for the prevention of type II diabetes.

Use Pace and Shape to look and feel better now and also to ward off diseases and disorders that may otherwise set in later.

Enhanced Performance

It's no secret that a healthy body will improve your performance in everything that you do. If you are stronger, you can carry groceries up a flight of stairs without a second thought. Strength training, specifically, will bring your cycling and overall productivity to a new level. Strength-trained men and women generally have better reaction times, increased flexibility and endurance, and leaner body mass than nonlifters. This makes everything easier, whether it's cycling up a hill or mowing the grass.

Strong muscles react more quickly than flabby ones. In the March 1994 issue of *Research Quarterly*, Roberta Rikli, PhD, professor of kinesiology, reported on a study of 44 women directed to hit a foot pad when a signal was given. Those with the strongest leg muscles reacted the fastest. This is due to the fact that toned muscles have more nerve fibers and blood vessels to help the impulse get from thought to action. This has strong implications for participants in any athletic competition, where reaction time often decides the winner.

The Pace and Shape program teaches you to take each muscle through a full range of motion, which improves your flexibility. As mentioned in chapter 6, increased flexibility can improve your performance and prevent injury both on and off your bike. Pace and Shape training also improves your muscular endurance. Improved muscular endurance helps you to endure a cycling race and also to move furniture for a long day at your garage sale.

If you are like most cyclists, you tend to neglect your upper body. You don't have the time or the inclination for the weight room. But

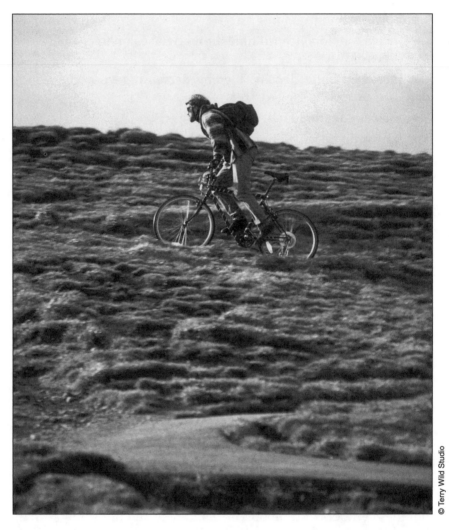

© Terry Wild Studio

If you strength train, you'll be able to get yourself (and your backpack) up that hill a lot easier.

if you do not stimulate muscle, you lose about six pounds of those precious fibers per decade. With less muscle, you burn fewer calories. You require less food, but if you eat the same, you gain fat.

Pedaling uphill hauling extra fat is tedious, but you can eliminate this burden by adding muscle instead. Muscle takes up less space than fat. One pound of fat bulges 18 percent more than a pound of muscle. In other words, fat occupies 1.1 liters per pound while muscle requires just 0.9 liters per pound. Therefore, if you lose fat but add muscle, you'll still become more compact and powerful. Making it up that hill will be a lot easier.

Muscle is the engine for your metabolism. So keep in mind that although more muscle improves performance and results in a faster metabolism, it also requires more food for energy. If you put on one pound of muscle, you must consume an extra 45 calories per day to support it. Therefore, you can eat more without gaining fat.

Creating a Pace and Shape Program

It is easier to adhere to a self-designed training schedule. Because Pace and Shape lends itself to individualization as your needs and goals change, you can develop your own Pace and Shape program, a program you will be more likely to stick with.

Prior to each workout, plan the order of your exercises and the intensity of your training. To avoid overtraining, on some days you should train until you cannot do another repetition, while on other days you should concentrate solely on perfect form. For best results, you should Pace and Shape two to four times a week with one day between sessions for your muscles to recover from the strength training component. Train each muscle group a maximum of twice a week. Just like Power Pacing, too many hard training days is catabolic (destructive) to your muscles and detrimental to your immune system, so straddle the fine line between a great workout and overtraining.

Use the strategies in chapter 4 to get you psyched up for each workout. Think of your goals and visualize your ideal self. Seconds prior to performing a set, visualize the groove you will take the weights through. Music can also be a great motivator, so select songs that will keep you going to the end of your workout. To maintain your focus, it's best to avoid working around phones, food, and children. If interrupted, make a note where you stopped so you can quickly resume your workout.

The Right Way to Train

To improve muscular endurance and cycling performance, work your large muscle groups in rapid succession using light weights. Lower repetitions and heavy weight build strength. After approximately five weeks you will have a stronger upper body, and you may notice muscle definition in your arms.

Perform one exercise per body part, doing a high number of repetitions with a weight you can comfortably control. Work the large muscle groups of the back and shoulders first, including your latissimus dorsi and your deltoids. Focus on one specific muscle group at a time. For example, to train your triceps, concentrate on the muscles in the back of your arm. Contract your triceps muscles on each repetition. Resist the weight in both the concentric (shortening) and eccentric (lengthening) phases of the movement.

Relax the rest of your body so a higher percentage of force is exerted behind your target muscle group. While working your target muscle, attempt to keep your facial muscles relaxed. You can yell if you want, but the rest of your body should rest.

Start with some easy repetitions to ease into your workout. Breathe normally during each exercise. Exhale during the contraction. Inhale on your short rests between each contraction. Imagine a surge of power as the blood enters the working muscle. Explode into each movement with a controlled yet 100-percent energized effort. Maintain good posture, keep your abdomen in, relax your neck, and keep your spine in a neutral position.

Power Point

Always move the weight through the full range of motion appropriate for each exercise. The amount of weight you lift should never dictate your form.

Perform one set of 10 repetitions at 60 percent of your maximum. Take about 30 seconds to finish each set. Your rest interval is the period between exercises. This recovery time should be minimal, including only the seconds required to change your form for a new range of motion. Your goal is to complete 10 repetitions of all 10 exercises with limited rest between sets.

Begin Pace and Shape slowly and progress gradually. Work up to doing Pace and Shape two to four times a week. Fortunately, if you were a former athlete, there is anecdotal evidence of muscle memory. Muscle memory implies if you were previously muscular, it will be easier to restore. For example, if you lifted weights in high school but have not touched a weight since, you may increase your muscle sooner than someone who has never previously trained with weights.

Always perform the shaping exercises after you have completed a cycling workout so you are already warmed up. (Make sure to stop pedaling before lifting the weights, and fully engage the resistance lever.) Furthermore, always finish with cool-down stretches for both the upper and lower body. (See chapter 6, pages 67-77.) Keep your Pace and Shape program simple, safe, packed with a variety of exercises, and fun!

Pace and Shape Exercises

If you have never strength trained before or if you are an older adult, Pace and Shape is for you. You can perform your Pace and Shape program without ever leaving your bike. All you need is a pair of dumbbells! Be sure you practice the following exercises with perfect form, and focus only on the muscle you are working during the last few repetitions. You may use association and dissociation techniques to help you through your Pace and Shape program, as discussed in chapter 4.

BENT-OVER ROW
Targeted areas: Latissimus dorsi, back

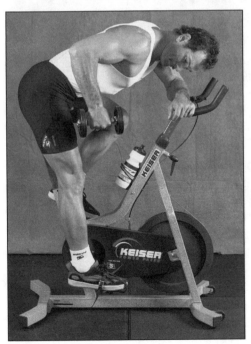

While bending from the waist, grasp a dumbbell in an overhand grip with your arm resting to your side. Keep your other arm securely on the handlebar using the forearm lean grip. Hold your torso parallel to the floor and pull the dumbbell up toward your chest, keeping your elbow close to your body. Maintain a flat back, and lower the dumbbell in a straight line back toward the floor. Repeat with your other arm.

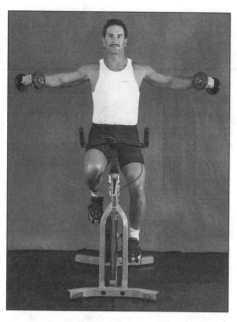

LATERAL RAISE
Targeted area: Deltoids

Sit with a dumbbell in each hand. Lead with your elbows as you lift them parallel to the floor, working the lateral aspect of your shoulders. Slowly raise your arms upward. The weight should provide tension in both directions.

MILITARY PRESS
Targeted areas: Deltoid, triceps

Remain on your saddle with good posture, holding the dumbbells on the back of your shoulders. With the dumbbells in an overhand grip, press them toward the ceiling as the resistance presses down. Keep your torso and head in a straight line with your chest out. Push with equal pressure from each arm upward to full extension. As you lower the dumbbells, keep constant tension in your shoulders.

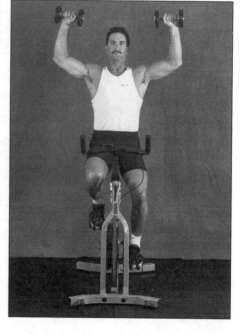

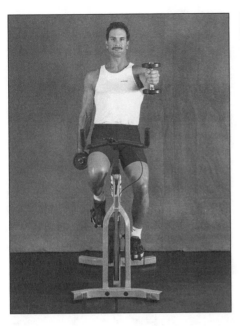

ANTERIOR RAISE
Targeted area: Shoulders

Grasp the dumbbells with your hands about shoulder-width apart, straight down at your sides with the palms facing each other. Keep your knees and elbows slightly bent and slowly raise the dumbbells one at a time, to shoulder height. Pause when your arm is parallel to the floor, and then slowly lower it back toward your thigh. Keep your shoulders back and down the entire time.

REVERSE CURL
Targeted areas: Forearms, biceps

Grasp the dumbbells at thigh level with an overhand grip, hands a little less than shoulder-width apart. Bring the arms up from the waist to shoulder level until your forearms touch your biceps. Lower the weights back down to your thighs using your elbows as the fulcrum or hinge.

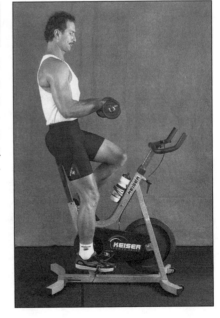

BICEPS CURL
Targeted area: Biceps

Grasp the dumbbells in an underhand grip, palms up, arms close to your sides. Allow the dumbbells to rest against your thighs. Pull the dumbbells toward your chin in a semicircle until your forearms touch your biceps. Keep your wrists locked. Lower the dumbbells on the same path you lifted them. Move the dumbbells up and down slowly through the full range of motion.

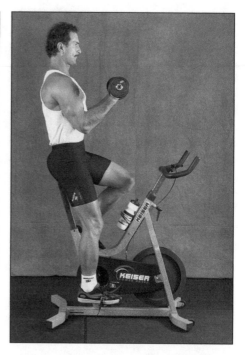

SHOULDER SHRUGS
Targeted area: Trapezius

Grasp the dumbbells with an overhand grip, palms down, your hands shoulder-width apart and your arms down to your sides. Keep your elbows straight as you droop your shoulders down as far as you can and then raise them back up as high as you can with the weight providing resistance in both directions.

Power Point

Imagine a surge of strength as the blood enters your working muscle.

TRICEPS KICKBACKS
Targeted area: Triceps

While one arm is in the forearm lean grip, grasp a dumbbell with your other hand and keep your elbow at a 90-degree angle. Extend your arm straight back until your elbow is locked. Hold for one second, then return to the 90-degree angle. After you finish a set, repeat with your other arm.

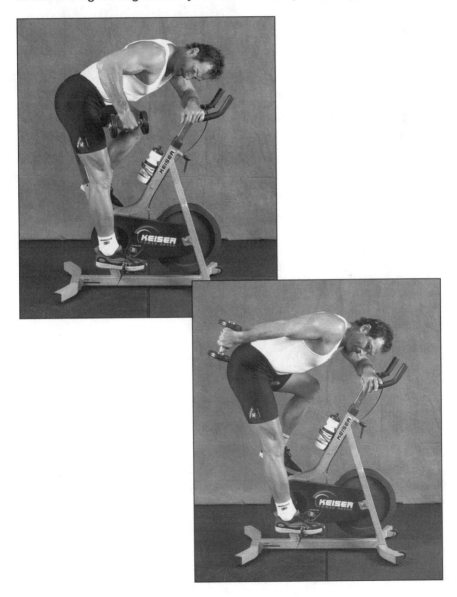

Power Point

Always finish with cool-down stretches for both the upper and lower body. (See chapter 6 for sample stretches.)

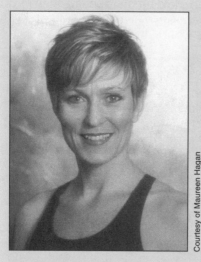

Courtesy of Maureen Hagan

Maureen Hagan's Pace and Shape Workout

As the education director for CanFitPro, a Canadian fitness professionals organization, I have very little time to strength train. When I know that I'm going to be very busy, I enjoy incorporating the shaping component at the end of a Power Pacing workout to ensure that I am maintaining the tone in my upper body. The following is a short workout I enjoy teaching.

After a three-minute recovery song consisting of the flushing and seated upright basic drills, apply full resistance to the bike, stop pedaling, and take your focus inside with a breathing drill. Sit upright and inhale through your nose for two counts and exhale out through your mouth for four counts.

The following exercises should be performed slowly, exhaling on the first movement, or concentric contraction, for one count and inhaling for three counts through the second movement, or eccentric contraction. Do 10 to 12 repetitions, increasing the number of sets to about three before moving on to the next exercise.

Using your handweights, do bent over rows, lateral raises, military presses, anterior raises, and triceps kickbacks in that order, as described in this chapter.

Upon completion of these exercises, take it to the floor and alternate 8 to 10 pushups with 20 abdominal crunches for two or three sets. Finish up with some gentle stretches for the upper and lower body found in chapter 6.

If you'd like to use the CycleSculpt exercises found in the next chapter, get out your Kris Kory Bike Band and do low rows, horizontal rows, side raises, anterior raises, front biceps curls, and triceps press-downs in that order. Again, do 10 to 12 repetitions, gradually increasing the number of sets. Begin each exercise using the purple band and progress to yellow so you always feel challenged.

Maureen is an international educator and fitness professional trainer. In addition to her worldwide travel as a trainer of fitness instructors, she brings physiotherapy training and 15 years of teaching to her expertise in lifestyle and sport performance programming. She is a Canadian-sponsored Three Stripe Athlete with Adidas and Bodylife Europe's International Educator of the Year for 1996.

Boosting Your Intensity

In one month, your body will have adapted to your Pace and Shape program. To continue to stimulate muscle growth, add intensity to your workout. Increase the weight, number of sets, or repetitions; or decrease your rest time between sets. Listen to your body. If your muscles are growing stronger and more flexible and you are not gaining additional body fat, you are doing everything right.

You may feel a burning sensation in your muscles as you increase your intensity. Soon you will anticipate the burn. The lactic acid burn and muscle fiber fatigue are signs that you are approaching muscular failure. Reaching muscular failure is difficult because you must endure some discomfort. One way to get your body to accept discomfort is to attend to the muscle group you are working. Another way is to dissociate yourself from the pain, as discussed in chapter 4. Try using a combination of both techniques: during your first few repetitions, dissociate by thinking about your upcoming set; however, during your final repetitions, focus on your muscles growing stronger and more powerful. Increasing strength is your measure of success.

If you reach a strength plateau, change your Pace and Shape program by doing one or more of the following:

- Modify the sequence of your routine.
- Perform different exercises.
- Change the range of motion of each lift.
- Increase your intensity.

- Upgrade your diet.
- Sleep more.
- Decrease the frequency of your workouts.

Although you should start out slowly, resistance training must be done with progressively higher intensities to increase strength. Use both high repetition/light weight and low repetition/heavy weight combinations to stimulate the different combinations of slow-twitch and fast-twitch muscle fibers.

Your muscles will adapt to heavier weight over time. Gradually increase the amount of weight you are lifting. Be patient. Do not work a muscle if it is sore from a previous workout. As you increase the weight, you will increase strength. For maximum strength gain, include sets of six repetitions. Each repetition should be intense enough that you reach exhaustion by the sixth. Maintain your muscular endurance by continuing your high repetition/low weight Pace and Shape workout.

A stronger body is a healthier body. Pace and Shape increases your strength, muscular endurance, and metabolism. You'll not only feel better, you'll look and perform better. The key to success is training smart. Upon reaching your strength goals, less intensity is required to maintain your fitness, but Pace and Shape should still be a part of your complete Power Pacing program.

You may be forced to curtail your Pace and Shape program due to an emergency or priority, but do not quit altogether. As little as one Pace and Shape workout each week can stimulate your muscle fibers enough to remain toned. Therefore, once you start Pace and Shape, don't quit—motivation to begin again may not come easily. A week's vacation is acceptable, but taking a month off means starting over. A prolonged break can lead to bone and muscle loss equivalent to several years of aging. It is easier to stay in shape than it is to get there. Use it or lose it is a true phenomenon.

Feel free to use dumbbells as described in this chapter, or substitute the same exercises using the Kris Kory Bike Band, which will be thoroughly explained in the next chapter. If you are short on time, the CycleSculpt resistance program (also explained in the next chapter) combines interval cardiovascular training with strength exercises all in a short 45-minute workout.

CYCLE-SCULPT

CycleSculpt was developed to provide the indoor cyclist stationary bike exercise intervals and strength training all in one workout. If you want to save time and are not able to spend a full hour working out doing a Pace and Shape program, this program can be used as a substitute, or it can be done on its own three or four times a week with a day or two between to recover. CycleSculpt differs from Pace and Shape in that the strength training components are done in intervals with cycling throughout the entire workout rather than just at the end. It combines basic and athletic drills with strength training exercises using the Kris Kory Bike Band by Spri Products, Inc.

The benefits of CycleSculpt include:

- increasing your $\dot{V}O_2$max—the rate at which your muscles efficiently use nutrients from oxygen (you will also be able to work out at a higher percentage of your $\dot{V}O_2$max because you will increase your anaerobic threshold);
- burning more total fat and calories in a shorter workout session, thereby maximizing the use of your time;
- stimulating both upper and lower body muscle fibers;
- changing your interval routine to avoid overuse injuries;
- spicing up your workouts; and
- allowing for a gentle break-in period since you are not cycling the entire time (making CycleSculpt a great class for beginners).

As with Pace and Shape exercises, to improve muscular endurance, work your large muscle groups in rapid succession. Do not dawdle between exercises. If you rest too long, you may lose "the pump" and decide to quit for the day.

Adding Variety to Your Workouts

CycleSculpt allows you to add variety to your strength training program. The strength portions of this program have set time intervals, such as 30 seconds or two minutes. The following five methods will help you organize your exercises and maximize muscle usage during your workout.

1. **Individual muscle isolation:** Working one muscle group with one exercise at a time

   Benefits: This is a great method to use when you have a very short interval and you want to maximize the fatigue of one specific muscle group. It is very focused and very intense.

   Example: Lateral raises to work the deltoids

2. **Pre-exhaustion super set:** Performing two different exercises in succession for the same muscle group

   Benefits: This method allows you to work more muscle fibers in one muscle group by changing the range of motion and still focusing on the same muscle group.

   Example: A lateral raise followed by a front raise to work the deltoids

3. **Super set:** Working two opposing muscle groups in succession

   Benefits: This method is another great time saver. Since muscle groups work in pairs, you can fatigue two opposing muscle groups within one interval.

   Example: Biceps curls for the biceps followed by triceps press-down for the triceps

4. **Tri-set:** Performing three different exercises in a back-to-back fashion in order to exhaust a specific area of the body

   Benefits: During longer intervals you are able to exhaust an entire area of the body by performing many exercises.

   Example: A seated low row, straight arm press-down, and horizontal row with the elbows level with the shoulders, all to exhaust the back muscles

5. **Giant set:** Performing four or more different exercises back-to-back in order to exhaust a specific area of the body

Benefits: Again, you are able to exhaust an entire part of the body by performing many exercises for the same area.

Example: A reversed standing lunge, standing donkey kick, hip extension, and hip extension with external rotation, all to work the posterior portion of the upper leg

CycleSculpt provides the training variety that muscles need to maximize results. The next section describes how to add more variety by moving to different counting patterns and downbeats of your favorite tunes.

Music and Motions

When you listen to music, you may tap your foot on a specific accent, or downbeat, of the music. The natural inclination to tap down on a downbeat demonstrates that our bodies automatically contract to certain rhythms.

Counting Beats

The deepest bass rhythms you hear are generally the downbeats of the music. These downbeats are usually put together in groups of eight. The group or phrase will often start with a heavier accent; this is where you would start counting from one and continue through eight if the music is made up of eight-count phrases.

Most dance or club music follows this eight-count pattern. If this is something you cannot feel right away, practice until it becomes more automatic. Use music that has 100 to 130 beats per minute. To determine the beats per minute of a song, count the number of downbeats in 30 seconds and multiply the number you get by two. See pages 86-87 and 92-93 for a few recommended music selections.

Contracting on the Downbeat

Performing the specific type of contraction you are emphasizing (concentric or eccentric) on the heaviest accents of the music will help you control your form and give you a guideline to follow when exercising. Here are a few examples:

1. Perform a biceps curl, focusing on the concentric (or shortening) portion of the contraction on the 1 count of each phrase and focusing on the eccentric portion of the contraction for the 2, 3, 4, 5, 6, 7, and 8 counts of the phrase. This will give you a very quick

concentric movement with a longer emphasis on the eccentric, or lengthening, phase.

2. Perform two biceps curls within eight counts by focusing on the concentric portion of the contraction on the heavy accents of 1 and 5. The eccentric phases of the contraction will happen on the 2, 3, 4 counts and the 6, 7, 8 counts. The main duration of the contraction will still happen on the eccentric phases, but the concentric phase is becoming a bit more focused. In order to stay with the music, you may have to shorten your range of motion to maintain proper body alignment.

3. Perform four biceps curls focusing on the concentric portion of the contraction on the heavy accents of 1, 3, 5, and 7. The main focus is now on the concentric portion of the contraction with hardly any emphasis on the eccentric phase. Your range of motion has become very short with a small peak contraction focus.

Keys to Using the Kris Kory Bike Band

When performing any exercise, it is important to use proper form. Remember to always maintain a neutral, stable spine by keeping the shoulders back and down, keeping the abdominal area strong and firm, and maintaining a slight natural lumbar curve in the back. Refrain from tucking the hips under or arching the back. Perform all exercises slowly with control first and then progress to quicker, more peak contraction-type movements if you prefer. That way, you'll have good concentration on the muscle group you wish to fatigue.

Power Point

Proper prepositioning of the body in each exercise is crucial to the success of working the desired muscle group most efficiently, thereby reducing the risk of injury.

When using the Kris Kory Bike Band, you should always maintain a straight line between your forearms, wrists, and palms. It is very common to break at the wrist when the exercise gets challenging, so maintain your focus.

The band provides three levels of difficulty. The dark band is the easiest, next is the light band, and most difficult would be to hold both tubes at the same time. See figure 11.1. If you are stretching the tubing more than three times its natural length, you should probably be using a more difficult band. Inspect your band from time to time for any tears or rips.

In conclusion, if an exercise is uncomfortable for your back, neck, or another part of your body, reposition, modify, or don't do it. Not all exercises are appropriate for everyone.

Positioning Yourself on the Bike

There are numerous ways you will position your body when performing the 40 CycleSculpt exercises described in the next section. There are also a number of places on the bike where you will attach the bike band in order to do these exercises.

In the following chart, each letter represents the bike band's point of attachment on the bike, along with a corresponding body position. These letters are teamed up with the CycleSculpt exercise numbers to form the drills on pages 167-170. This way, for each exercise, you'll know exactly what body position you should maintain, as well as where the band should be attached to the bike.

For example, lets take a look at the second exercise in the Equal Time Speed Bursts drill on page 167. In "9A," the number 9 refers to

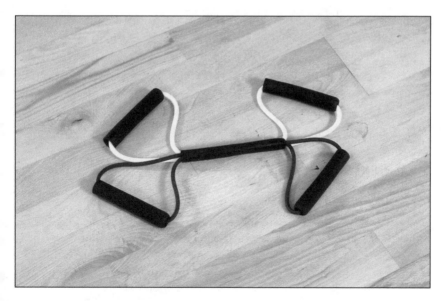

Figure 11.1   The Kris Kory Bike Band.

exercise 9 (Compound Low Rowing) on page 152. To find out what the "A" refers to, take a look at the chart below. Now when you get to the drills, you'll know exactly what exercise to do and exactly how to do it.

Keep in mind that there are many different ways you can position your body and many different places where you can attach the bike band for each exercise. Feel free to consult a Keiser master trainer and learn even more variations!

Band Attachment		Body Position
Place the center of the band...		
A	...around the handlebar stem.	Sit in the saddle and hold onto each handle with both hands.
B	...under the handlebar tightening pin.	
C	...in the triangular space shown in photo "C" on page 145.	
D	...under the seat post pin; hold onto the handles between your legs.	
E	...under the seat post pin; hold onto the handles outside of your legs.	
F	...over one of the aggressive grip positions.	Sit in the saddle and hold onto each handle with one or both hands.
G	...over one of the overhand grip positions.	
H	...around the top portion of one of the bike forks.	
I	...around the bottom portion of one of the bike forks.	Lie down in front of the bike with your knees bent and feet on the floor. The top of your head faces the back of the bike.

Band Attachment	Body Position
Place one handle of the band…	
J …over one of the aggressive positions.	Sit in the saddle and hold onto one handle of the band with one hand.
K …over the little front wheel on the front frame of the bike.	
L …under the seat post pin; hold onto each handle outside of the legs.	
M …over the outside of the back foot of the bike.	
N …over one of the overhand grip positions.	Stand behind the saddle and hold onto one handle of the band with one hand.
O …over the little front wheel on the front frame of the bike.	
P …over one of the overhand grip positions.	Stand facing the side of the bike and hold onto the handle of the band with one hand.
Q …over the little front wheel on the front frame of the bike.	
R …over the little front wheel on the front frame of the bike.	Stand next to the bike with one foot in the handle of the band.
Place both handles of the band…	
S …in a close overhand grip over the handlebars or keep the handles in your hands.	Sit in the saddle with the band around your upper back and under your arms.
T …in an aggressive grip over the handlebars or keep the handles in your hands.	

Illustrated Positions

The following are a few close-ups of the different places the bike band attaches to the bike. The letters refer to the chart on pages 142-143. Positions A-H, K, and M are illustrated. For a complete list, refer to the chart on the previous page.

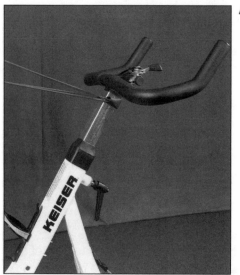

A

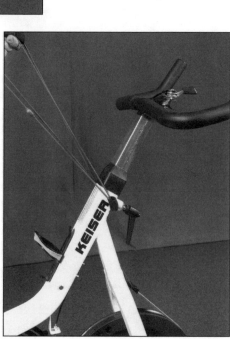

B

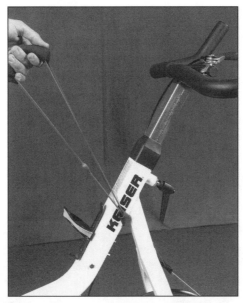

C

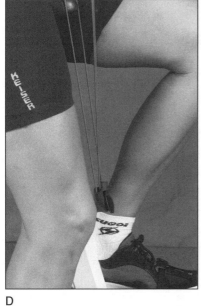

D

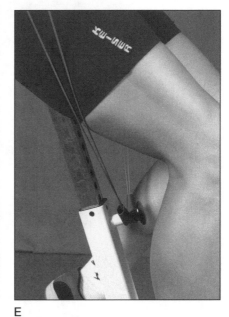

E

Power Point
Always remain seated when using the handlebar tightening pin to keep it stable, and never lean back.

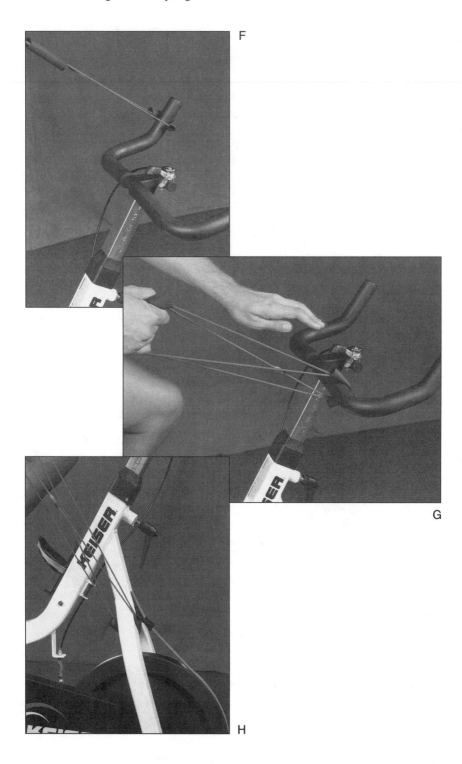

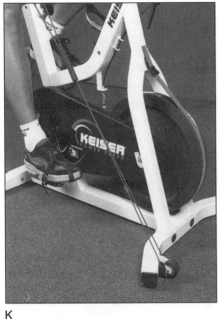

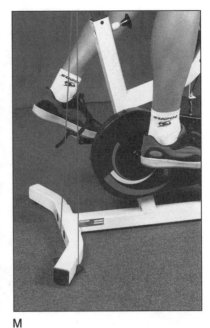

K   M

CycleSculpt Exercises

Each of the following exercises is numbered so that when you do the drills starting on page 167, you can quickly refer to the complete exercise description.

> **Power Point**
> Do not pedal when you are doing CycleSculpt exercises. Have the resistance tightened completely.

POSTERIOR REGION OF TORSO

The following exercises work the latissimus dorsi, rhomboids major and minor, teres major and minor, posterior deltoids, trapezius, and spinal erectors.

1 LOW ROWS

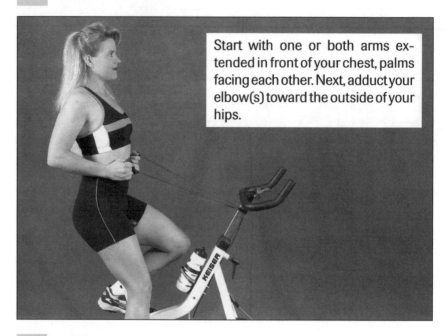

Start with one or both arms extended in front of your chest, palms facing each other. Next, adduct your elbow(s) toward the outside of your hips.

2 HORIZONTAL ROWS

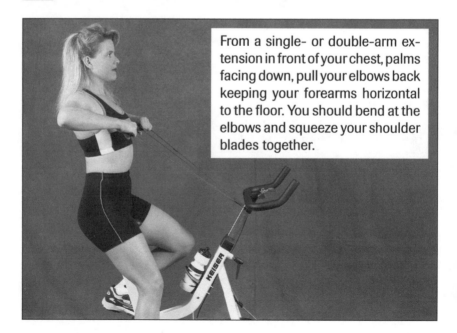

From a single- or double-arm extension in front of your chest, palms facing down, pull your elbows back keeping your forearms horizontal to the floor. You should bend at the elbows and squeeze your shoulder blades together.

3 STRAIGHT-ARM PRESS-DOWN

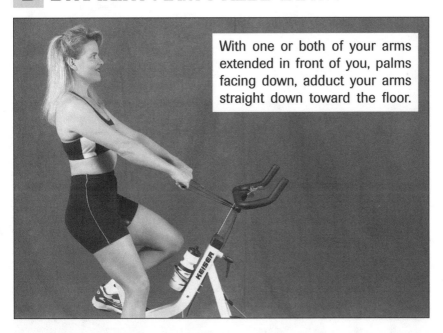

With one or both of your arms extended in front of you, palms facing down, adduct your arms straight down toward the floor.

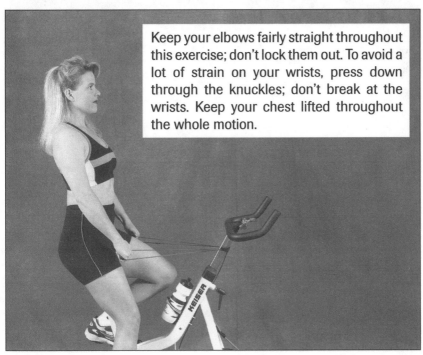

Keep your elbows fairly straight throughout this exercise; don't lock them out. To avoid a lot of strain on your wrists, press down through the knuckles; don't break at the wrists. Keep your chest lifted throughout the whole motion.

4 PULL-DOWN

With one or both of your arms extended above your head, palms facing away from you, adduct your elbow joints toward the side of the lower portion of your rib cage allowing your elbow joints to bend. This exercise can be done standing, bent at the waist, or lying supine behind the bike.

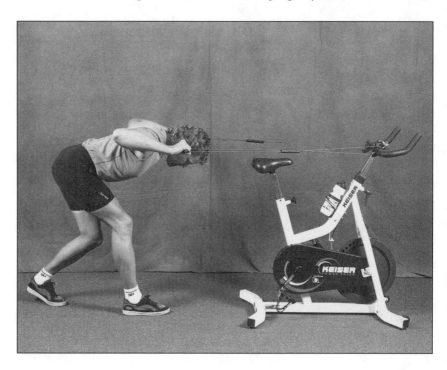

5 LOW BACK EXTENSIONS

Move from a neutral spine to a more extended position by moving from an aggressive riding position to a reversed basic riding position.

6 COMPOUND HORIZONTAL ROWING

With your torso in a vertical position, perform circular movements with your elbow. Keep your palms facing down and your forearms horizontal to the ground.

7 PULL-OVER

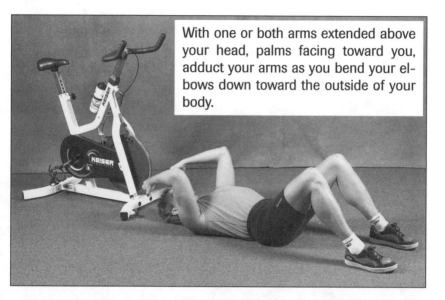

With one or both arms extended above your head, palms facing toward you, adduct your arms as you bend your elbows down toward the outside of your body.

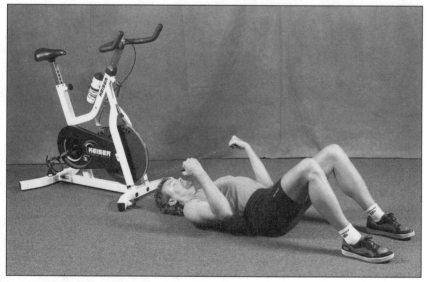

8 SHOULDER SHRUGS

With your arms at your sides, lift your shoulders up and down.

9 COMPOUND LOW ROWING

Keep your torso vertical. Starting with both arms extended out in front of you, perform circular movements with your elbows at the sides of your body with your palms facing each other and your elbows low.

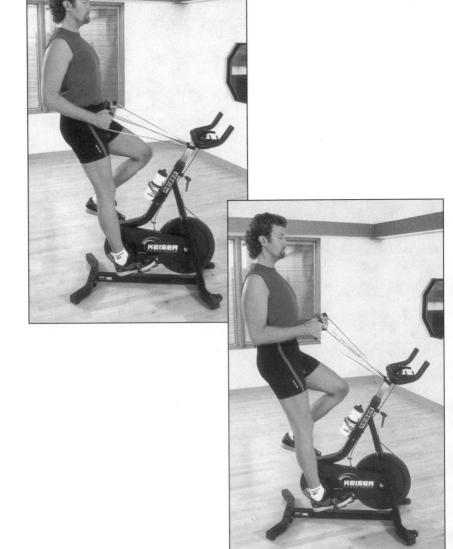

SHOULDER REGION

The following exercises work all regions of the deltoid area.

10 LATERAL RAISES

Start with your arms by your sides, then raise them out to the sides just below shoulder height. Lead with the back of your hand, being careful not to let your wrist bend. Keep your palms facing downward.

11 ANTERIOR RAISES

Start with your arms by your sides, then abduct one or both of your arms forward to shoulder height with your palms facing each other.

12 REVERSED FLY

With your arms extended out in front of you, palms facing each other, open one or both arms laterally, focusing on pulling your shoulder blades back and down. Keep your elbows slightly bent. Don't break at the wrist; lead with your knuckles and the back of your hand.

13 MILITARY PRESS

Hold your arms straight out to your sides, then bend your elbows to form two right angles in line with your shoulders. With your palms facing forward, extend your arms straight up. Press through your knuckles without breaking at the wrist.

14 INTERNAL SHOULDER ROTATION

Start with one or both bent elbows at your hips, palms facing forward. Internally rotate your shoulder by closing your hands toward each other. Keep your elbows at your hips.

15 POSTERIOR STRAIGHT-ARM RAISE

With your arms straight at your sides, your elbows slightly bent, your shoulders rotated in, and your palms facing back, lift one or both arms straight up behind you. Take care to keep your spine neutral.

16 EXTERNAL SHOULDER ROTATION

Start with one or both bent elbows at your hips, palms facing each other. Externally rotate your shoulder by opening your hands away from each other. Keep your elbows at your hips.

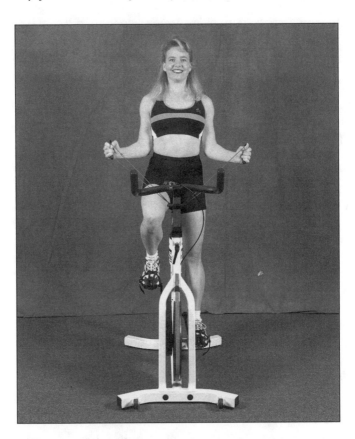

ANTERIOR REGION OF TORSO

The following exercises will work your pectoral muscles.

17 HORIZONTAL CHEST PRESS

Form a right angle with one or both arms parallel to the floor and positioned at shoulder height. With your palms facing down, extend your arms straight forward. Stand with your back facing the handlebars.

18 LOW- TO MID-LEVEL CHEST PRESS

Starting with one or both hands at hip level, palms facing toward each other, extend your arms straight forward ending at shoulder height. Stand with your back facing the handlebars.

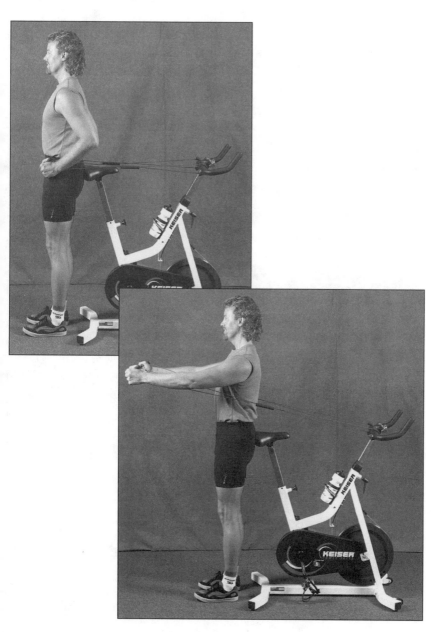

19 FLAT FLY

With one or both arms extended out to the side slightly below shoulder height, palms facing forward, adduct your arms toward the midline of your body in front of you, keeping them slightly below shoulder height. Keep your elbows slightly bent.

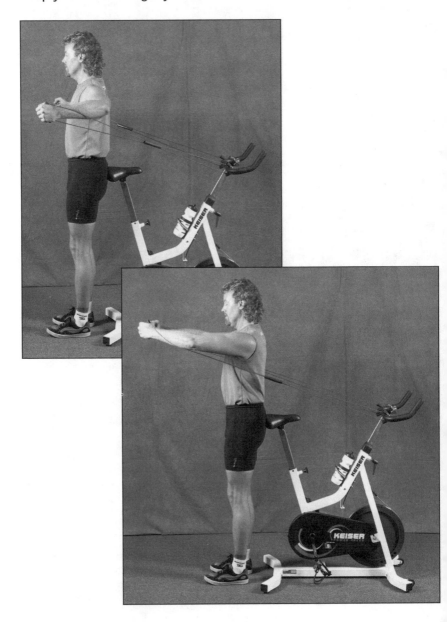

20 COMPOUND SCOOP

Start with both arms at your sides and palms facing away from you. Bring your hands toward each other, bending your elbows toward each other, scooping up, and finishing with the elbows and forearms together in front of you. Your elbows should be slightly below your shoulders.

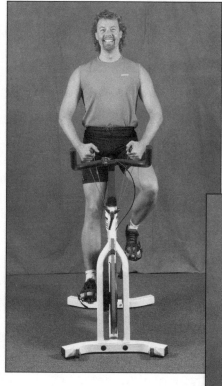

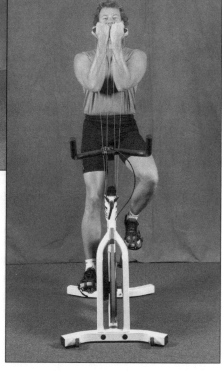

21 ARM PUSH-UPS

Start with a corner grip with elbows slightly out to the side. The band is around your upper back under your arms, and the handles are in the overhand grip position.

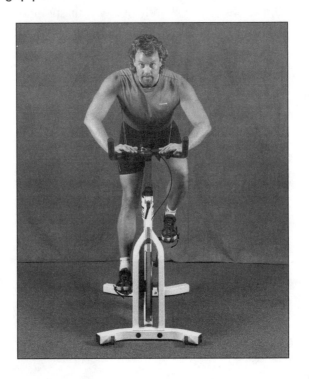

22 INCLINE FLY

With one or both arms extended out to the side slightly below shoulder height, palms facing forward, adduct your arms toward the midline of your body in front of you, keeping them slightly above shoulder height. Keep your elbows slightly bent.

23 DECLINE FLY

With one or both arms extended out to the side slightly below shoulder height, palms facing forward, adduct your arms toward the midline of your body in front of you, bringing them down toward your navel. Keep your elbows slightly bent.

24 CROSSOVER

This exercise uses the same motions as the other three fly variations except that you cross over the midline of your body with one or both arms at the same time.

UPPER ARM REGION

These exercises work the biceps brachii, triceps, brachioradialis, and brachialis.

25 FRONT BICEPS CURL

Start with one or both arms extended at your side with palms facing the front. Flex your elbow joints, bringing your forearms toward you.

26 SIDE BICEPS CURL

With one or both arms extended at your side, externally rotate your shoulder joint so that your palms face to the side. Flex your elbow joints, bringing your forearms toward your biceps.

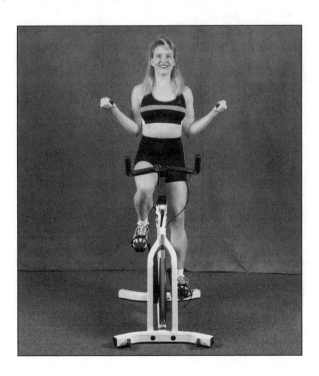

27 CROSS BICEPS CURL

With one or both arms extended at your side, your shoulder joints internally rotated, and your palms facing in, flex your elbow joint. This is the same as the front biceps curl except that your palms should face each other.

28 TRICEPS PRESS-DOWN

With one or both elbows at your sides, forearms parallel to the floor, palms facing down, extend your elbow joint. Make sure to press through your knuckles. Don't break at the wrist.

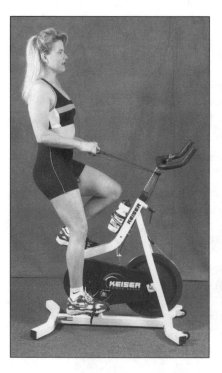 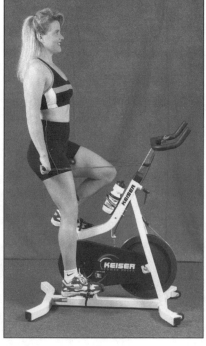

29 TRICEPS KICKBACK

With one or both bent elbows behind your back and your hands at your hips, extend your elbow joint as you press your palm behind you. Your shoulder joint should be slightly internally rotated.

3O OVERHEAD PRESS

To find the starting position, extend one or both arms above your head, then bend your elbows so they're right by your head and your hands are almost touching the backs of your shoulders. Extend your elbow joints, pressing your knuckles up toward the ceiling.

31 TRICEPS HORIZONTAL EXTENSION

Starting with the back of your hand in the center of the chest and your elbow at shoulder height, palm facing out, extend your elbow joint to the side, keeping the whole arm parallel to the floor.

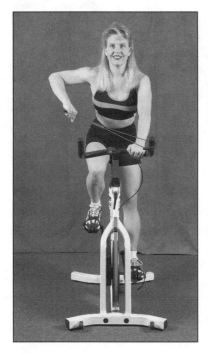
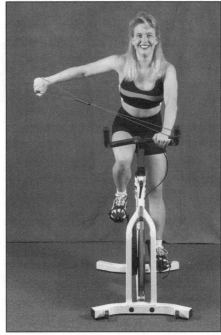

MIDSECTION

The following exercises work the rectus abdominis and obliques.

32 FRONT CURL

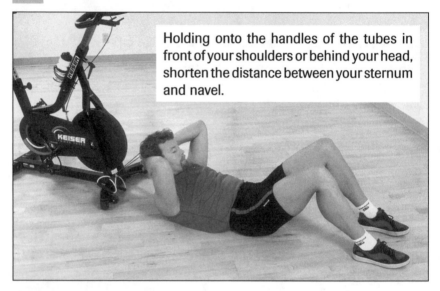

Holding onto the handles of the tubes in front of your shoulders or behind your head, shorten the distance between your sternum and navel.

33 OBLIQUE

Holding onto the handles of the tubes in front of your shoulders, behind your head, or both on the same side for more resistance, move diagonally, imagining sliding one side of your rib cage into the other hip pocket.

Power Point
Never sacrifice proper form or technique for an exercise.

BASIC LEG EXERCISES

These exercises work the gluteus, hamstrings, quadriceps, and calves. Use two bands for these exercises. For leg exercises 34, 35, 38, and 39, stand next to the bike with both of the handles over the handlebars in overhand grip and the other handles on the moving foot.

34 STANDING DONKEY KICK

Starting with your knee up toward your waist, extend your leg down and slightly to the rear. The band should be on the foot farthest from the bike.

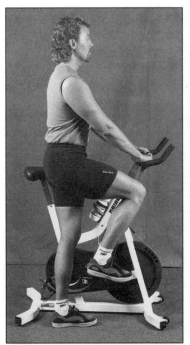
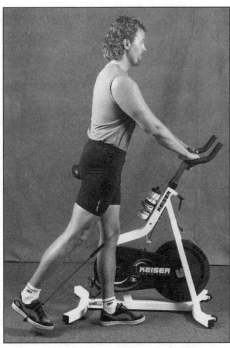

35 HIP EXTENSION

With a straight leg, press it back taking care not to stress your low back. The band should be on the foot farthest from the bike.

36 CALF RAISES

With straight legs, raise up onto the balls of your feet.

37 HIP ADDUCTION

Stand facing the side of the bike with one leg (the working leg) slightly in front of the other. Adduct the working leg toward and in front of the standing leg. Move the working leg with a slight bend in the knee.

38 EXTERNAL HIP ROTATION

With a straight leg extended behind you, rotate out at the hip socket without moving your pelvis. Your leg should be the only thing that moves; keep the rest of your body braced. The band should be on the foot farthest from the bike.

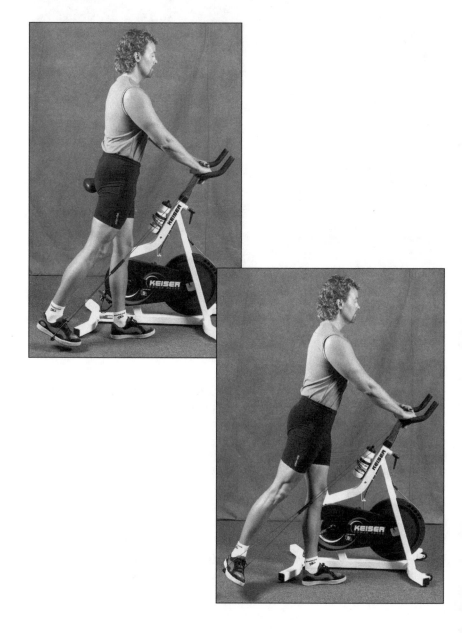

39 HIP ABDUCTION

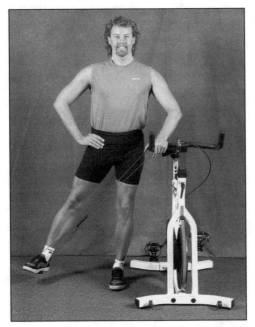

Stand next to the bike with one leg slightly in front of the other. Abduct the working leg (outside leg) laterally. Move the working leg to the side with a slight bend in the knee.

40 REVERSED SINGLE LUNGE

Stand next to the bike. This time the stationary leg is the leg you are actually focusing on. Slide the opposite leg behind you as if you were going to kneel down. At the end of the back movement, you should have a right angle in each leg. Make sure your front knee is directly over or behind your front heel. Keep your chest up. For an extra challenge two handles may be placed on the front working leg and the other handles should be held in the arm on the same side of the body as the working leg.

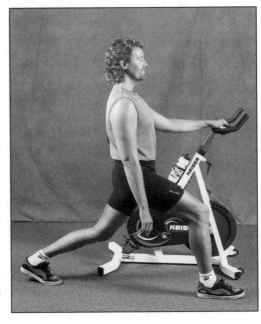

Joint Preparatory Movements

Now that you've been introduced to all of the CycleSculpt exercises, it's time to get your body ready for a full-blown CycleSculpt work-out. After completion of the regular cycling warm-up found on pages 63-67, it is important to do joint preparatory movements. These are slow, controlled movements with resistance. Move the upper body as if moving through peanut butter or heavy mud. Feel the joint areas getting hot. In the following combinations do not use a band, just keep the muscles very taut.

Combo 1

1. With your arms at your sides, circle your wrists back and around.
2. Rotate your shoulders back and around.
3. Lift your elbows up, back, and around.
4. Backstroke with both arms.
5. Reverse the direction of 1 through 4.

Combo 2

1. Extend one or both arms straight up and reach for an imaginary pull-down bar. Next, pull your arms down, resisting as you move.
2. With your arms forming right angles at your sides and your elbows level with your shoulders, imagine you are squeezing a big ball between your elbows and forearms. Contract your chest and the front of your shoulders as you squeeze your arms toward each other and then resist as you go back to the starting position.
3. Starting with your arms extended out at your sides, perform a decline fly exercise, allowing the forearms to cross each other. Then pull your elbows back up to the side again where you started.
4. Starting in a military press position with your arms forming right angles at your sides and your elbows level with your shoulders, internally rotate and then externally rotate your shoulders.

Combine combos 1 and 2 into one fluid motion and finish with some gentle upper body stretches.

CycleSculpt Drills

When planning your CycleSculpt workouts, plan to work all the major muscle groups in the body during your strength intervals. Following are several athletic drills with ideas on how to incorporate the strength segments into them. Combine the following drills in the sequence written or mix and match them in an order that you prefer.

In the following drills, the first column gives you the order in which the exercises should be performed. The second column presents the name of the basic or CycleSculpt exercise. The third column represents the body position and / or bike band position you will use. Lastly, the length of time you should do each exercise is given.

Equal Time Speed Bursts

#	Exercise	Position	Time
1	Fast hammer	Basic riding position	30 sec.
2	Compound low rowing	9A (p.152)	30 sec.
3	Fast hammer	Aggressive riding position	30 sec.
4	Compound horizontal rowing	6A (p.150)	30 sec.

"A" means that the bike band attaches just under the handlebars.
Repeat this drill twice.

Speed Play Variation

#	Exercise	Position	Time
1	Low rows	1B (p.148)	30 sec.
2	Horizontal rows	2B (p.148)	45 sec.
3	Straight arm pressdowns	3B (p.149)	25 sec.
4	Reversed flys	12B (p.153)	20 sec.

"B" means that the bike band attaches just under the handlebars tightening pin.

Incorporate the above four exercises into a speed play format that lasts 4 to 10 minutes. Speed play requires you to select basic drills and frequently change the time you spend in a basic drill, your body position, your hand position, your speed, and/or resistance. Add the above exercises between intervals of your choice.

Pyramid Climb Variation

#	Exercise	Position	Time
1	Posterior straight-arm raises	15K (p.153)	15 sec.
2	Fast hammer	Seated basic riding position	15 sec.
3	Front biceps curl	25K (p.159)	30 sec.
4	Standing climb	Basic riding position	15 sec.
5	Combine posterior straight arm raises and front biceps curls.	15K and 25K (pp.153 and159)	45 sec.
6	Standing climb	Aggressive riding position	15 sec.
7	Combine side biceps curls, posterior straight arm raises, and front biceps curls.	26K, 15K, and 25K (pp.153 and159)	60 sec.
8	Standing climb	Basic riding position	15 sec.
9	Combine triceps press-downs and triceps kickbacks.	28N and 29N (p.160)	45 sec.
10	Fast hammer	Seated aggressive riding position	15 sec.
11	Triceps horizontal extensions	31N (p.161)	30 sec.
12	Fast hammer	Seated basic riding position	15 sec.
13	Alternating cross biceps curls	27N (p.160)	15 sec.

"K" means one handle of the band is placed around the little front wheel on the front frame of the bike.

"N" means one handle of the band is placed over one of the overhand grip positions.

Hill Sprints Variation

#	Exercise	Position	Time
1	Seated climb	Basic riding position	10 sec.
2	Standing climb	Basic riding position	10 sec.
3	Fast hammer	Seated basic riding position	10 sec.
4	Lateral raises	10B (p.153)	30 sec.
5	Repeat 1-3		
6	Combine anterior raises and external shoulder rotations.	11B and 16B (pp.153 and 154)	30 sec.
7	Repeat 1-3		
8	Combine lateral raises, anterior raises, and external shoulder rotations.	10B, 11B, and 16B (pp.153 and 154)	30 sec.
9	Repeat 1-3		
10	Combine military presses and lateral raises.	E13 and E10 (p.153)	30 sec.

"B" means that the bike band attaches just under the handlebar tightening pin.

"M" means that one handle of the bike band attaches over the outside of the back foot of the bike. Use two bands, one for each hand.

Long Hill Sprint Variation

#	Exercise	Position	Time
1	Standing climb with lead leg emphasis on the right leg	Standing climb position	30 sec.
2	Reversed single lunges	40 (p.165)	10-15 reps.
3	Standing donkey kicks	34P (p.163)	10-15 reps.
4	Hip extensions	35P (p.163)	10-15 reps.
5	External hip rotations	38P (p.164)	10-15 reps.
6	Standing climb leading with the right leg	Standing climb position	30 sec.

"P" means that one handle of the bike band attaches to the overhand grip position and the other attaches to your foot.

Only one leg is worked per set.

Repeat with the other leg, starting with the lead drill on the left leg.

Always finish your CycleSculpt workout with cool-down stretches for all the major muscle groups in the body, as found in chapter 6.

CycleSculpt can provide you with lots of variety, and the Kris Kory Bike Band, with three different levels of strength abilities, can give you the challenge you need. Mix your intervals up and try not to get stuck doing the same thing the same way all the time. Remember, variety is what your muscles need in order to change. They will get used to the same workout quickly, and you won't see the results you are looking for.

Enjoy your CycleSculpt workouts. These workouts are fun to do either alone or with a friend as well. Have your friend act as your personal trainer, timing the cycling interval drills for you and telling you what sculpting exercises to do. Then switch places and you can train your friend. Watch each other's form and make sure the shoulders are always back and down and the wrists remain neutral. Oh yeah, and don't forget to breathe!

TAKING IT TO THE ROAD

Even if you have the most prolific Power Pacing instructor or the most reliable Power Pacing partner, sometimes you need a change. Consider moving your workouts back to the great outdoors. Cycling outdoors reveals sights not seen by even the average motorist. Admire bucks, does, and birds of all shapes and feathers. Scenic cycling tours build muscle, trim fat, increase endurance, and improve your cardiovascular power. If you enjoy Power Pacing, you will appreciate the challenge of outdoor cycling.

Power Pacing drills can enrich your outdoor experience. Perform a rhythmic dip drill under a tree limb. Pedal into headwinds using your aerodynamic aggressive riding position. Stand up on a long hill sprint up a mountain. Air up your tires, trade your towel for a helmet, and fill your water bottles. Ride in pairs, join tours, or compete in races. Outdoor cycling has a wide range of physiological demands. From 200-meter sprints to the ultra-endurance Race Across America, your body can adjust to 100-degree temperatures, mountains, and gusty headwinds. Fear not. Power Pacing strengthens you to handle these challenges and more.

Elite cyclists discipline their bodies and minds. There are no timeouts, substitutions, or coaching sessions during competition. Cyclists spend hours alone with their thoughts. Draw upon your Power Pacing drills to shape your outdoor cycling.

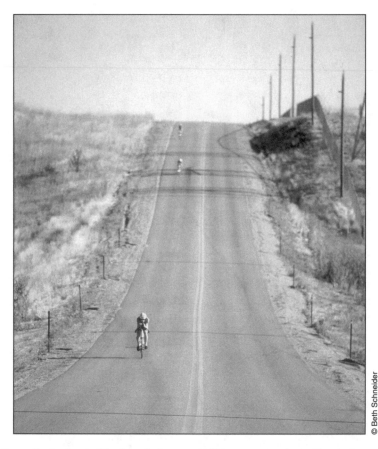

© Beth Schneider

Use Power Pacing's mind/body techniques to help keep you motivated for the long, solo rides.

Ready for Outdoor Cycling

Road and off-road cycling uses a variety of muscle groups. Quadriceps, hamstrings, gluteals, calf muscles, and upper body muscles propel you up hills and into hurricane headwinds. Power Pacing trains these muscles. Each Power Pacing drill is different: standing climbs require standing on the pedals for long uphill climbs, and speed bursts are quick, impulsive bursts of speed as though making a break from a pelaton. And because you recruit muscle groups in patterns, they are toned, strong, and ready long before your first race of the season.

The Race Across America and other endurance events require a variety of body positions using different muscle groups. Lean over leg is similar to ice skating on a bike. When you perform lean over leg, your muscles are recruited in a pattern similar to that of actually pedaling up a hill. Power Pacing in the aggressive riding position teaches you to hold a tight, streamlined posture for hours. These exercises and positions enable you to tolerate hours on your aerobars in endurance events.

The discipline Tom gained from Power Pacing enabled him to finish the Race Across America. Endless revolutions per minute (rpms) of Power Pacing prepared him for the interminable boredom of pedaling through the Midwest. Power Pacing's wet sport ambience equipped him for the stifling California desert. And while other racers succumbed to saddle sores, pedaling on his Power Pacer made outdoor cycling a treat.

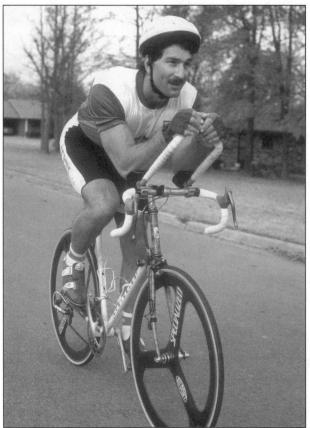

Courtesy of Tom Seabourne.

Power Pacing prepared Tom Seabourne for the grueling Race Across America.

Power Pacing also familiarizes you with short stretches of training, just below your anaerobic threshold. But sometimes you must "go anaerobic." Whether dashing up a hill or sprinting to finish a 20-mile tour, you feel lactic acid. This requires a physiological adjustment. Power Pacing improves your ability to tolerate lactic acid. Speed drills, such as pedaling at nearly maximum exertion from five seconds to two minutes, improve your anaerobic capacity. Your anaerobic capacity determines your ability to break away from the pack, climb steep mountains, and sprint to the finish of a race. You learn when to surge and back off your pedaling. This improves your road racing abilities, ultimately delaying the onset of fatigue.

Some studies suggest that there may be a correlation between 30-second speed bursts at near maximum capacity and outdoor cycling performance. A significant similarity was demonstrated between power output on 30-second intervals and actual performance during racing. Faster riders also showed more structure in their training than slower riders. Thus, interval training on your Power Pacer and a preplanned total body workout will help you succeed in competition.

Making the Most of What You've Got

Whether you are a rotund endomorph, skinny ectomorph, or muscular mesomorph, you can take Power Pacing to the road. If you are heavy, you will work harder on climbs, but you will sail past other riders on your descent. Skinny riders are generally robust on the uphill. And muscular men and women can power their bikes through 30-mile-per-hour headwinds.

Speed and Endurance Fibers

Your Power Pacing muscles need sugar and mind-to-muscle stimulation to turn your pedals. Your goal is to activate as many quadriceps, hamstring, gluteal, and calf muscle fibers as possible during each Power Pacing program. Flushing may recruit only half the number of muscle fibers of a fast hammer. One motor neuron may innervate 1,000 muscle fibers in your calf during a seated climb, while another motor neuron may activate 10,000 muscle fibers in your gluteals during a standing climb.

You have two basic types of muscle fibers: Type I and Type II. Your postural muscles are Type I, endurance, red, and are considered slow-twitch fibers. These muscles balance you in an erect position while pedaling. Type I fibers are recruited during the first few minutes of Power Pacing. They are capable of less force but help you pedal longer than Type II fibers do.

Successful competitive road racers possess both fast- and slow-twitch muscle fibers. If you boast a predominant number of fast-twitch fibers, you probably prefer to turn your pedals more quickly. These fibers are more efficient at fast contraction speeds. Racers who have a preponderance of slow-twitch fibers or who have a large cross-sectional area of muscle prefer pushing bigger gears at a slower rate. For some, this slower contraction causes blood to occlude in vessels. Oxygen demand exceeds oxygen supply, forcing them to use anaerobic processes. Lactic acid increases, and the removal rate is lessened. Premature fatigue may result. To avoid premature fatigue, switch to an easier gear and pedal faster. Your goal is to move the bike forward as fast as it will go using as little energy as possible. In Power Pacing, however, you want to use as much energy as possible to recruit more muscle fibers and increase your aerobic power.

> At 2:00 A.M. during the Ironbutt, Tom and another competitor were vying for first place. They were averaging 27 miles per hour while racing side by side. Tom was in his large chainring, requiring him to pedal slow, steady, powerful strokes. His rival's pedals were flying, but he took frequent coasting breaks. Different riders have different cadences. Tom and his challenger were pedaling just below their anaerobic thresholds at their best power-to-speed ratio to maximize their genetic potential.

Type I, slow-twitch fibers use oxygen, which means they are aerobic in nature. They are smaller and contain less energy than Type II fibers, but their blood-oxygen content is high, providing for greater endurance over long events. They provide endurance for your 45-minute Power Pacing workout. Slow-twitch fibers can contract repeatedly without fatigue. They are used during endurance events.

Type II, fast-twitch fibers are recruited for fast, powerful speed bursts. There are two subclasses of Type II fibers. Type IIb fibers are nonoxidative (not aerobic). They are faster, stronger, and provide more force for a 15-second sprint finish, but they fatigue quickly. A fast hammer for 15 seconds at a perceived exertion rating of 20 uses Type IIb fibers. Type IIb fibers are anaerobic with a high glycogen content and fast-twitch rate. They have few capillaries and low endurance but a high power output.

> A rival tried to pass Tom during the Race Across America. Tom boosted his speed by about two miles per hour. This increased intensity was just below his anaerobic threshold. Tom was barely holding on, but he increased his speed once more by recruiting Type IIb fibers. He kept up for a while, but soon he crossed over his anaerobic threshold and felt the lactic acid burn. He depleted all of the energy in his muscles, and for the next 10 miles he floundered until the lactic acid was recycled to be used for energy. His adversary pedaled out of sight. If Tom would have kept a steady pace, just below his anaerobic threshold, he would not have bonked. (*Bonk* is a cycling term which means that all of the sugar in your muscles has been used up.)

Type IIa intermediate fibers are somewhat oxidative. They use a combination of the aerobic and glycogen systems. These are re-

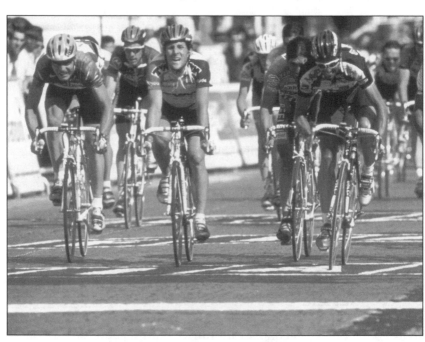

Their fast-twitch fibers help these cyclists sprint to the finish.

cruited after Type I fibers. Type IIa intermediate fibers are fast-twitch with moderate myoglobin content, capillary density, force production, and endurance. They are slightly trainable. You can prepare them to be like Type IIb fast hammer speed fibers or Type I long hill climb endurance fibers.

If you do interval training, your Type IIa intermediate fibers will take on the characteristics of sprint fibers. Long, slow distance endurance training, however, will move them toward the Type I, slow-twitch, red, oxidative fibers. Type I fibers are used during your warm-up while pedaling at between 0 and 25 percent resistance. As you increase to 50 percent resistance, Type IIa intermediate fibers kick in. And, finally, when you take the resistance to 75 percent and increase your speed to a fast hammer, you fire up your Type IIb fibers.

Power Point

In your Power Pacing workouts, you can concentrate on fast-twitch or slow-twitch fibers, depending on which style of outdoor riding you prefer.

Power Pacing uses all of these fiber types in a 45-minute workout. If you want to become a good all-around cyclist, simulate an all-terrain workout. Practice powering up imaginary hills and forging through long straightaways against a strong headwind. Your ultimate goal is to use Power Pacing to increase your aerobic power and recruit all of your muscle fibers to make you a better cyclist.

Training Your Muscle Fibers

To train both slow- and fast-twitch fibers, add resistance to the flywheel, simulating a long hill sprint. When you reach the top of the imaginary hill and approach your anaerobic threshold, your slow-twitch fibers fatigue and your lactic acid rate skyrockets. Click your resistance dial down a few notches and fast hammer down the other side of the hill. In a few moments your fast-twitch fibers fatigue and a new cycle begins.

Elite cyclists turn their pedals between 90 and 110 rpms. It is neuromuscular—a mind/body thing. Your mind must recruit the correct muscle fibers and fire them in the correct sequence to keep you pedaling fast. Keep your feet soft on the pedals. Let speed come. The harder you try, the more slowly you pedal. When you feel as if you are about to lose control, remember that your feet are secured to

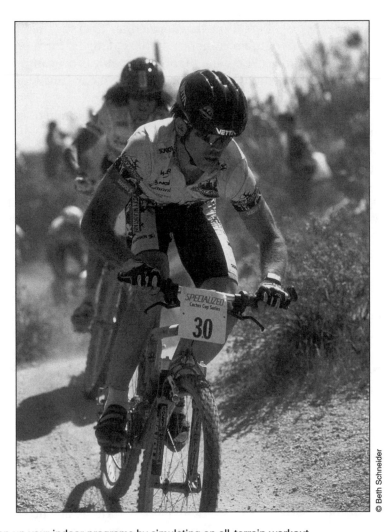

Liven up your indoor programs by simulating an all-terrain workout.

the pedals. Your knees are like pistons. Allow your legs to fly. Amaze yourself at how briskly you pedal.

> Tom is cursed with predominantly slow-twitch fibers. Ninety miles into a century race, Aaron, a teammate, whispered that they should break away from the pack. Aaron signaled a sprint and took off. He was already 100 feet ahead before Tom's slow-twitch fibers finally reacted. Tom realized that if he wanted to win, he would have to make a break early in the race. Or he would have to find races longer than 100 miles.

Competition Tips

Train the same way you compete. Concentrate. If you are tempted to skip training, remind yourself that you are a competitive cyclist. Work on yourself a little bit each day during your training. Become more relaxed, more focused, more fun-loving. If you have trouble concentrating, imagine that you are racing.

Just before your race, ask yourself what could be so important to cause you to waste half your day fretting. Understand that every cyclist gets butterflies. Take a deep breath from your diaphragm and relax muscles that feel tense. Visualize yourself appearing comfortably focused and prepared for your cycling performance. When your imagined cycling performance begins, "see" everything going as planned. Imagine a glitch in your cycling, but see yourself smiling, recovering fully and completely. Be spontaneous.

Your relaxation will allow you to be more flexible, providing for a better cycling performance. Don't focus so much on yourself. Other people don't care as much about you as you do. Empathize with the anxiety of your cycling companions. Help relieve their burden by relaxing. Take control of yourself. Be brave.

When your event begins, see yourself as graceful and powerful, fast and strong, flexible and tenacious, cool and spontaneous, invincible, a finisher. Don't try so hard. Relax. Smile when you feel anxious. Breathe from your diaphragm if something excites you.

When you find yourself dwelling on a mistake, laugh it off. If something bothers you, ask yourself why; then fix it. If you can't fix it, don't let it bother you. Say key words to yourself, such as *relax* and *focus*. Let it flow. But get pumped: be enthusiastic, vigorous, alert, and energetic. Focus on the present. You will lose your concentration now and then during a long race, so prepare for it and let it go. Let a real or imagined crowd spur you to your best ride.

No matter how bad things get during a race, remember that your opponents, like you, have two legs—they can be beaten. If you race opponents who are faster than you, be smarter. Even if you have to slow your pedal stroke and push big gears, no one cares who looked better when a race is on the line. Sometimes you must take risks to win, yet become detached from the results. There is always another race.

Now that you know how Power Pacing prepares you for outdoor cycling and you're ready to take it outdoors, contact the following organizations for more information on cycling groups in your area:

- Your local chamber of commerce
- Your local recreation center
- Your local community college
- The United States Cycling Federation (USCF)
  One Olympic Plaza
  Colorado Springs, CO 80909-5775
  719-578-4949
- The Ultra Marathon Cycling Association (UMCA)
  Box 53
  Canyon, TX 79015
  806-499-3210

Power Pacing indoors is fun, but for a change of scenery, outdoor cycling can't be beat. Wear a helmet, carry a water bottle filled with a beverage of your choice, and begin pedaling. Pedal to your favorite imaginary Power Pacing tunes, but leave your walkman at home. Use your pedal stroke to recreate the beat. Use a rearview mirror to keep a lookout for traffic coming up from behind. Finally, perform regular maintenance on your bike for years of outdoor fun.

HOME TRAINING

Power Pacing at home is easy and convenient. No gyms or instructors are necessary. Home training is designed to provide you with a safe and effective routine to keep your skills sharp and, more importantly, to motivate you to sustain a training regimen. A consistent pedaling program can help you Power Pace into your twilight years. Grab a towel, fill your water bottle, cue your favorite cassette tape, and rock and roll.

Power Pacing at Home

Most home exercise equipment usually becomes a coat rack or clothesline. Your Power Pacer is different. Although it is a single machine, you can do a variety of programs on it. You do not need a spotter, so it is safe to train by yourself. And you can customize your workout to meet your needs at any moment.

Preparing for Your Workout

As always, mentally prepare yourself for a rigorous Power Pacing session. Imagine the feel of an awesome workout. "See" yourself as having achieved your Power Pacing goals. Allow no interruptions! Take the phone off the hook and lock the doors. This is your practice time. While you are preparing to begin, if thoughts such as "I can do this later" or "I don't have time for this" enter your mind, see a big red stop sign and remember your Power Pacing goals. A full-length mirror can be helpful for checking your form. Make sure that you have easy access to water.

Your Workout Begins

Step 1: Begin Power Pacing with a six- to eight-minute warm-up as discussed in chapter 6. Watch yourself in a mirror and let your thoughts drift to your goals.

Step 2: After the warm-up, continue pedaling and stretch out the upper body to limber up. Hold each stretch for 15 to 30 seconds. It will help you to relax. At the same time imagine your muscles as rubber bands.

Step 3: When you hear the next song, perform the first Power Pacing warm-up drill of your choice.

Step 4: Now that you are warm, get ready for your first high-intensity Power Pacing drill of your own choosing. Perform each drill for the duration of a song. Each song lasts approximately three to five minutes.

Step 5: Cool down with flushing and stretching.

Step 6: Close your eyes and visualize having reached your Power Pacing goals.

Home Intervals

When you do not have time for a full-blown outdoor workout, try Power Pacing home intervals. Speed bursts or hill sprints can replace long, slow distance pedaling. Spend six to eight minutes warming up at an easy pace. Then gradually increase your intensity until you are pedaling at about 70 percent of your maximum speed. You may feel a slight burn in your legs. Your lungs may open up for the first time in years. Hold this pace for about a minute. Then slow to your steady state tempo for two minutes. Increase your speed again to 70 percent for another leg-exploding, lung-expanding minute. Repeat these intervals several times. Cool down to a relaxed pace for another five minutes.

Power Point

A suggested training interval for a hardcore athlete might include riding hard for 15 minutes at a pace you can barely maintain, then flushing to recover. Add one 15-minute interval each week until you reach three work intervals.

Mindless Home Training Program

When you just want to listen to some good music and you don't want to make the effort to watch the clock for a pyramid climb, simply do speed play. Although you are all alone in your exercise room, imagine you are about to begin the Race Across America. Create the race, moment by moment, and depending on how you feel, push yourself and then back off. The race begins and ends in your mind. Set an alarm clock for 45 minutes and let the microcosmic race begin. When the gun goes off, you sprint to the front of the pack. Rest for a few moments and then attack your first hill by adding heavy resistance to the dial. Fast hammer down the other side of the hill with light resistance and then push steadily into a headwind with moderate resistance on your dial. When your alarm goes off, raise your arms in victory. Then cool down and stretch.

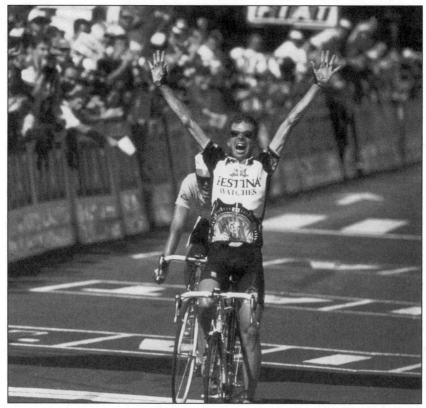

© Beth Schneider

Imagine yourself in a race. You've won!

Home Video Dissociation Training

Point your Power Pacer toward your television. Turn on your ceiling fan, take a sip of water from your water bottle, and insert a videocassette into your VCR. Television movies do not work as well because of commercials. If you have a choice, watch an action/adventure movie. Warm up for six to eight minutes while the credits are rolling at the beginning of your flick. Your steady-state easy pedaling and posture breaks will occur during slow parts of the movie, while the plot thickens. But when the action heats up, so do you. Your goal is to increase your intensity by speeding your cadence or adding resistance during the most exciting parts of the show. Before you know it, you will have Power Paced twice as long as your normal 45-minute workout. Be sure to cool down and stretch.

Tips on Home Training

Training at home should always be performed as if you were being observed by an instructor. Maintain perfect posture and perform all of your body positions with precision. It is easy to forget about form if no one is watching. For this reason it is a good idea to supplement your home training with an occasional Power Pacing workout in the gym.

1. Concentrate on your training without distraction.
2. Practice specific drills that work for your goals and temperament. You may prefer Race and Pace drills over rhythmic drills if you are a competitive cyclist striving to improve your aerobic power.
3. Work on weaknesses you might not normally practice in front of others.
4. Practice to music to develop rhythm and enhance endurance.
5. Your fitness gains depend largely on the intensity of your training.
6. If you get tired and sloppy, slow down or take a break.
7. Sip water between songs.

For some, it is difficult to drink during exertion. Drinking on the bike is an art. Power Pacing teaches you to prime the pump by forcing yourself to sip fluids. A rule in Power Pacing is to drink before you are thirsty. Your thirst mechanism may malfunction during Power Pacing. Body weight may drop a few pounds before you feel parched.

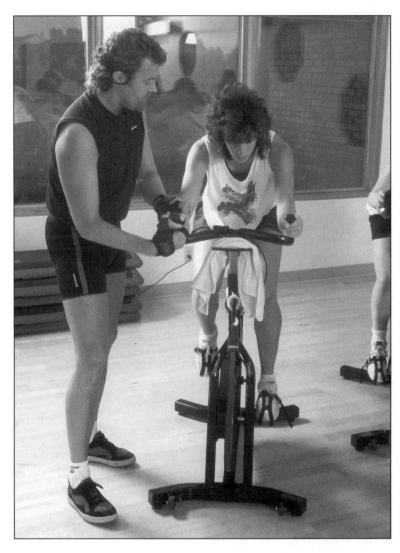

Train at home like you've got an instructor looking over your shoulder. Perfect form is a must!

When you lose significant water, your blood cannot carry glucose and oxygen to your muscles as effectively.

The Final Stretch

Home workouts can improve your in-the-gym Power Pacing performance and your outdoor cycling experience, or they may simply be an end in themselves. Maintaining perfect body position and controlling your intensity are key ingredients to your Power Pacing home workout success. You will improve your fitness and cycling performance if you follow the step-by-step programs provided in this book. Cycling can lift the spirit. Whether Power Pacing or cycling out in the rain, pedaling is revitalizing. Set a goal and begin pedaling. Endorphins carry your body further than you ever dreamed. Your body is busy churning while your mind is free. You control the speed, the tempo, and the resistance. You decide if you want to succeed and when it's time to quit. You are the master on your bike.

Benson, H. 1984. *Beyond the relaxation response*. New York: Times Books.

Benson, H. 1987. *Your maximum mind*. New York: Times Books.

Benson, H. 1993. *The wellness book*. New York: Simon & Schuster.

Borysenko, J. 1988. *Minding the body, mending the mind*. New York: Bantam Books.

Burke, E. 1986. *The science of cycling*. Champaign, IL: Human Kinetics.

Burke, E., and Newton, H. 1983. Improved cycling performance through strength training. *National Strength and Conditioning Association Journal* 5(3), 6–7, 70–71.

Csikszentmihalyi, M. 1994. *Flow: The psychology of optimal experience*. New York: Simon & Schuster.

Edwards, S. 1993. *The heart rate monitor book*. Port Washington, NY: Polar Electro.

Dossey, L. 1993. *Healing words*. New York: Harper Collins.

Freidman, M. 1989. A master of moving meditation. *New Realities*, June, 11–20.

Goleman, D. 1993. *Mind body medicine*. Yonkers, NY: Consumer Reports Books.

Iknoian, T. 1997. A New Spin on Indoor Cycling. *Fitness Matters* 3(6), 1–4.

Kory, K. 1997. *Keiser Power Pacing instructor training manual*. Fresno, CA: Keiser Corporation.

Langer, E. 1989. *Mindfulness*. New York: Addison-Wesley.

Rikli, R. 1994. *Research Quarterly*, March.

Seabourne, T. G. 1996. *Cross-training*. Dubuque, IA: Eddie Bowers.

Seabourne, T. G., Weinberg, R. S., and Jackson, A. 1981. Effects of visuo-motor behavior rehearsal, relaxation and imagery on karate performance. *Journal of Sport Psychology* 3(3), 228–238.

Seabourne, T. G., Weinberg, R. S., and Jackson, A. 1985. Effect of arousal and relaxation instructions prior to the use of imagery. *Journal of Sport Behavior* 6, 209–219.

Wilmore, J., and Costill, D. 1994. *Physiology of sport and exercise*. Champaign, IL: Human Kinetics.

Kristopher Kory has been certified by the American Council on Exercise (ACE) for more than a decade and is an international exercise and fitness workshop presenter. He is the North American Education Director for Keiser Corporation and is the co-developer of the Keiser Power Pacing programs, along with fitness authority Karen Voight. He has certified over 5,000 new cycling instructors to teach the Keiser Power Pacing programs.

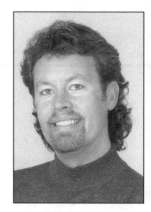

Kory has more than 16 years of aerobic, dance, fitness programming, and club management experience. He's been featured in and/or has authored over 50 publications and is the creator of Keiser's new cycling videos "Power Pace and Shape" and "Race and Pace." Kory has also been featured on Fox News with his own segment, "Fit Tip of the Week." He is a popular speaker at fitness conferences, including those of the International Dance and Exercise Association and Club Industry. Kory lives in Naples, Florida.

Tom Seabourne, a PhD recipient in exercise science, currently holds four Ultra Marathon Cycling Association (UMCA) world records and finished in the top ten in the Race Across America (RAAM). He is a two-time U.S. National Heavyweight Taekwondo Champion and was runner-up in the World Taekwondo Championships. He also is an accomplished tennis competitor.

Certified by the ACE and the American College of Sports Medicine, Seabourne is a master trainer for Keiser Corporation's Power Pacing Programs. He also serves as a consultant with the Topper Sportsmedicine Group in Vail, Colorado. He has written five books and over 200 articles on sport topics. He writes a weekly fitness column, "Your Personal Trainer," for the *Longview News Journal* and enjoys promoting fitness on his weekly radio call-in talkshow, "Total Fitness," and his

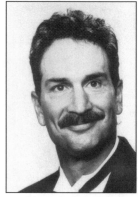

website, **www.onlinetofitness.com.** Seabourne lives in Mt. Pleasant, Texas, with his wife Danese and five children: Alaina, Grant, Laura, Susanna, and Julia.

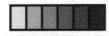

FITNESS SPECTRUM SERIES

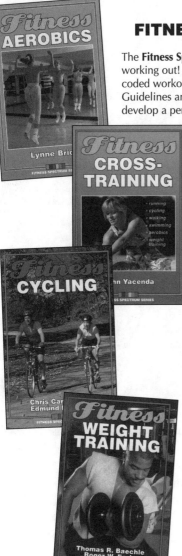

The **Fitness Spectrum Series** takes the guesswork out of working out! Each book is packed with easy-to-use, color-coded workouts that will add variety and produce results. Guidelines and sample programs are provided to help develop a personalized training program.

Fitness Aquatics
Item PCAS0963 • ISBN 0-87322-963-0
$15.95 ($21.95 Canadian)

Fitness Aerobics
Item PBRI0471 • ISBN 0-87322-471-X
$14.95 ($20.95 Canadian)

Fitness Walking
Item PIKN0553 • ISBN 0-87322-553-8
$15.95 ($21.95 Canadian)

Fitness Swimming
Item PHIN0656 • ISBN 0-88011-656-0
$17.95 ($26.95 Canadian)

Fitness In-Line Skating
Item PNOT0982 • ISBN 0-87322-982-7
$15.95 ($21.95 Canadian)

Fitness Stepping
Item PPIL0835 • ISBN 0-87322-835-9
$14.95 ($20.95 Canadian)

Fitness Cross-Training
Item PYAC0770 • ISBN 0-87322-770-0
$14.95 (19.95 Canadian)

Fitness Weight Training
Item PBAE0445 • ISBN 0-87322-445-0
$15.95 ($21.95 Canadian)

Fitness Cross-Country Skiing
Item PGAS0652 • ISBN 0-88011-652-8
$15.95 ($21.95 Canadian)

Fitness Cycling
Item PCAR0460 • ISBN 0-87322-460-4
$14.95 ($20.95 Canadian)

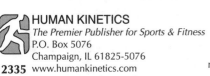

HUMAN KINETICS
The Premier Publisher for Sports & Fitness
P.O. Box 5076
Champaign, IL 61825-5076
2335 www.humankinetics.com

To place your order, U.S. customers call
TOLL FREE 1-800-747-4457.
Customers outside the U.S. place
your order using the appropriate telephone
number/address shown in the front of this book.

No other stationary bike takes you this far.

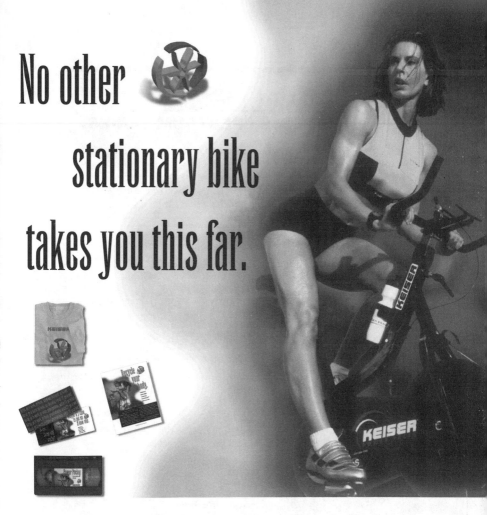

It takes more than talk to make a great bike program. At Keiser, we combine leadership in product quality and research with the knowledge and celebrity appeal of Karen Voight to give you cycling programs you'll be proud to offer.

There's *Power Pacing*™, a 40-minute musical ride that strengthens glutes, quads, hamstrings and calves while melting fat and building stamina. Pace and Shape combines a heart-pounding cardio with light body sculpting. *Race and Pace*™ takes riders to the fringes of speed and endurance. And our newest program, *FreeWheeling*, uses a non-fixed gear bike to add a fourth dimension to indoor cycling.

Our programs are good enough to sell themselves. We help you anyway — with banners, posters and ads on a ready-to-print CD. Plus training manuals and videos, and a maintenance video to help keep you rolling. All against a backdrop of a national PR campaign that spreads the news about *Power Pacing*™ and *FreeWheeling* to attract new members. And a personal on-site instruction option that brings certification and continuing education credits right into your facility.

Find out how easy it is to break out of the pack by calling Keiser today at **1-800-888-7009.**

Nobody takes you farther than we do.

KEISER®
Performance you can bank on.™

KEISER CORP.
2470 S. Cherry Ave.
Fresno, CA 93706 USA
1-800-888-7009
Tel: (559) 256-8000
Fax: (559) 256-8100
http://www.keiser.com